the
food
medic
for life

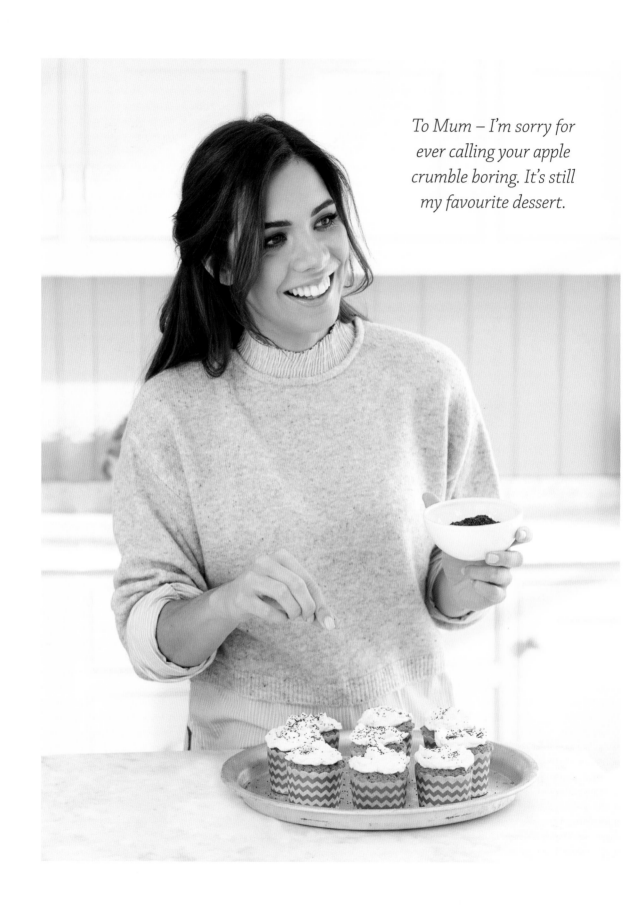

To Mum – I'm sorry for ever calling your apple crumble boring. It's still my favourite dessert.

DR HAZEL WALLACE

the
food
medic
for life

Easy recipes to help
you live well every day

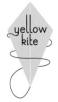

First published in Great Britain in 2018 by Yellow Kite,
an imprint of Hodder & Stoughton
An Hachette UK company

1

Hardback ISBN 978 1 473 65057 2
eBook ISBN 978 1 473 65055 8

The advice herein is not intended to replace the
services of trained health and fitness professionals, or
be a substitute for medical advice. You are advised to
consult with your health care professional with regards
to matters relating to your health, and in particular
regarding matters that may require diagnosis or medical
attention.

Colour origination by BORN

Printed and bound in Italy by L.E.G.O. S.p.A.

Hodder & Stoughton policy is to use papers that are
natural, renewable and recyclable products and made
from wood grown in sustainable forests. The logging
and manufacturing processes are expected to conform
to the environmental regulations of the country of
origin.

Yellow Kite
Hodder & Stoughton Ltd
Carmelite House
50 Victoria Embankment
London EC4Y 0DZ

www.yellowkitebooks.co.uk
www.hodder.co.uk

Publisher: Liz Gough
Senior commissioning editor: Tamsin English
Project editor: Natalie Bradley
Copy-editor: Trish Burgess
Art direction and design: Hart Studio
Photographer: Ellis Parrinder
Food stylist: Jordan Bourke
Props stylist: Louie Waller
Senior production controller: Susan Spratt

Note on nutritional information

The nutritional information was calculated by a registered
dietitian using Dietplan 6 dietary analysis software. It is
an estimate only and may vary depending on the brand of
ingredients used, and due to the natural biological variations
in the composition of natural foods such as meat, fish, fruit
and vegetables. It does not include the nutritional content of
garnishes or any optional accompaniments recommended for
taste/serving in the ingredients list.

Where not specified, ingredients are analysed as average
or medium, not small or large. All recipes were analysed
using 65g (2.3oz) eggs. Readers should consult their doctors
before altering their diet, particularly if they are on a set diet
prescribed by their doctor or dietitian.

The information and references contained herein are for
informational purposes only. They are designed to support,
not replace, any ongoing medical advice given by a healthcare
professional and should not be construed as the giving of
medical advice nor relied on as a basis for any decision or
action.

Fibre analyses were obtained by a registered dietitian using
the AOAC method, the method that manufacturers are
required to use by law to declare fibre on packaged foods.

Low-sugar recipes contain less than 5g sugar per 100g and
low-salt recipes less than 0.3g salt per 100g. Values specified
by the Food Standards Agency.*

The glycaemic index categories (low, medium, high) listed
for each recipe are estimates only and were calculated by a
registered dietitian. The GI values of each ingredient were
sourced from the International GI Database and proportions
of carbohydrate contributing to the total value of each recipe
calculated in order to determine the GI value of the recipes. If
an ingredient did not have a published GI value, the GI value
of the most similar foodstuff was used as a substitute. For
this reason, and the fact that food preparation and cooking
methods can affect a food's GI value, it is possible that some
of the recipes may produce a higher or lower blood glucose
response than predicted from the estimated GI rating listed.
It is recognised that the most accurate method would be
to test each recipe once made, but without lab conditions
we have used this method to offer you some guidance.
Therefore, it would be beneficial for people with diabetes to
monitor their own blood glucose responses to the recipes
in order to determine which ones produce the lowest blood
glucose responses.

* Food Standards Agency. (2005 [updated 2010]). Eat Well
– your guide to healthy eating: 8 tips for making healthier
choices. [PDF] Available at: www.food.gov.uk/sites/default/
files/multimedia/pdfs/publication/eatwell0708.pdf

CONTENTS

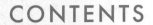

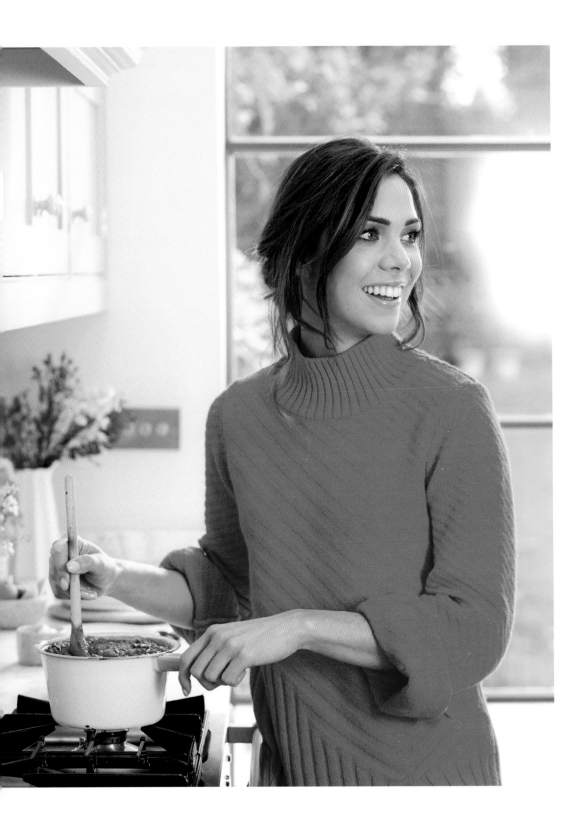

INTRODUCTION

Food has always been an integral part of my life. I was raised in a seaside village called Blackrock in County Louth on the east coast of Ireland. As kids, my sisters and I were involved in the cooking process from a young age, doing anything from picking fruit in the orchard for apple pie to peeling the spuds for Sunday's roast dinner. It was common for the whole family to have some role in the mealtime ritual, especially at dinnertime when we were all home from school and Dad was back from work. My mum would call us all to the table and we wouldn't think to argue – even if it meant leaving whatever game we were playing in the garden. We would always invite our friends in as we knew Mum always set an extra place and popped an extra potato in the pot just in case. Dinnertime became my favourite part of the day because it was when we were all together, discussing what we'd done, telling jokes and sharing stories – all while enjoying a home-cooked meal.

When I was fourteen years old, my most cherished part of the day became my worst nightmare when my dad had a stroke at the dinner table. It was a Saturday afternoon and Dad had been out cutting the grass, just as he always did at the weekend. We sat down to one of his favourite meals, spaghetti bolognese, but he struggled to lift his fork to his mouth and his arm fell limp beside him. At the hospital he was diagnosed with a transient ischaemic attack (TIA), which is sometimes called a mini-stroke. He was not an unhealthy man, but shortly before the TIA he had been diagnosed with high blood pressure and type 2 diabetes. He was advised to watch his sugar intake and exercise regularly, and although I remember him checking his blood sugar every morning, I'm not sure how much nutritional advice he was ever given by his GP.

Unfortunately, that mini-stroke was just the beginning of something much more sinister, and later that week he had a bigger stroke that took his life.

Everything I associated with dinnertime – love, family and happiness – was lost. I stopped sitting at the dinner table, and soon I stopped eating too. I was just too sad and too angry to pretend things were the same. My weight plummeted as grief consumed me. Eating became a chore, something I knew I had to do, but I didn't want to.

My road to recovery began when I asked my GP to refer me to a dietitian. I knew what I needed to do to get myself well again, but I felt like I couldn't do it alone – or at least lacked the energy for it. My mum came with me to my first consultation and greeted the dietitian with tears rolling down her cheeks, moved to see that it was the same person who'd been involved in my dad's care while he was in hospital following his initial stroke.

With a structured plan and weekly weigh-in targets to meet, I found a glimmer of hope inside me. Week by week I grew stronger, both mentally and physically, simply by eating again. I returned to a healthy weight within four months and found myself back in the kitchen, helping Mum with the cooking and sitting down with the rest of the family at dinnertime.

FOOD AS MEDICINE

Losing my dad was the hardest experience I have ever gone through. I will never fully get over the grief, but his death and my reaction to it taught me a very powerful lesson. I learnt first-hand how food can be a double-edged sword, acting as a driver of disease, but also as a conduit for good health.

Now, as a doctor, it has become even more apparent to me that what we eat can have huge implications for our health, both positive and negative. I come across lifestyle-related diseases, such as type 2 diabetes, heart disease, stroke and dementia, on a daily basis, and I witness the frustration and dissatisfaction of both patients and healthcare providers at the management of these conditions. There is a huge disconnect between conventional medicine and nutrition, and that space has been filled largely by unqualified voices who obscure any meaningful advances in understanding how nutrition influences health.

Chronic diseases such as stroke and heart disease are the largest causes of morbidity (illness) and mortality, not to mention the largest healthcare expense, in the developed world. Sadly, medicine as we know it is doing a pretty poor job of addressing these problems, and it seems that we are fighting a losing battle.

Don't get me wrong – I am so grateful for the advances in modern medicine and I prescribe medication daily in my practice. If it weren't for vaccinations and antibiotics, most of us would be dying from relatively trivial ailments such as urinary tract and chest infections. The advances in conventional medicine are incredible, often like something from sci-fi movies: we can reattach limbs, restore sight to the blind, and even perform complex surgeries with robots.

However, the diseases people suffered from and died of in the 1900s are very different from 21st-century 'killers'. Whereas infectious diseases once saw off most people, it's self-inflicted chronic diseases such as obesity and diabetes that do the job today.

I don't think there is a quick solution to present-day problems, but I do think we need to shift our mindset from sick care to health care. We need to create a new healthcare model that involves both patients and doctors working together not only to prevent and treat disease, but to maximise health.

We can't bury our heads in the sand and pretend that food doesn't matter to our health. We can't simply prescribe a pill for every ill. There isn't always a cure, but we have a good shot at prevention if we take the right steps now.

I went into a lot of detail about nutrition in my first book, *The Food Medic*. I am passionate about this subject and think it's really important for everyone to have a basic understanding of food so that they can make their own informed choices about it. After all, what we put into our bodies determines how we function.

Food is family, it's friends, it's comfort, it's home, it's tradition, it's life-giving, it's celebration, it's therapeutic, it's love, it's health. Let's not forget this.

FOOD IS MORE THAN NUTRIENTS

In my early twenties at university, I tried my fair share of faddy diets in a bid to shed the stubborn few pounds I had gained from my sedentary, fast food-fuelled lifestyle. Food was my comfort when I was homesick or stressed with exams, but it was simultaneously my enemy. Food became just another thing on the to-do list, another thing to stress about. I soon became bored with dieting and, frustrated at my results – or lack of them – decided to do a bit of research. I immersed myself in papers on nutrition and health, and began to apply what I had learnt in the literature to my own life. I started cooking from scratch, with as many wholefood ingredients as possible, using the basic skills I had picked up from my mother and grandmother. My meals were not time-consuming or fancy in any shape or form, and, most importantly, they weren't restrictive. I was eating a balance of all nutrients (carbs, fats, proteins) and choosing better-quality foods.

On reflection, it wasn't just *what* I ate that changed, but *how* I ate and thought about food. I reconnected with both food and cooking, and didn't falter (despite my busy schedule) because I had finally learnt to respect my body enough to feed and nourish it with real, wholesome food.

In fact, what and how we eat is important for everyone. It plays a central role in the cultural identity of any nation and shapes our relationship with food. It defines us.

The kitchen is generally the heart of the home. Across cultures and time, the very act of sharing a meal is a universal expression of friendship; it embodies values of hospitality, gratitude, sacrifice and compassion. The shared meal is an opportunity not only to nourish ourselves with food, but to create and strengthen our bonds of family and friendship, to teach and learn.

Given that food is central to our lives, I believe we should have a better understanding of it. However, industrialisation, travel and tourism, technology and media, and our fast-paced lives have led us to become oddly disconnected from our food. I fear we often overthink what we eat, arguing about it, restricting or over-indulging in it, analysing and dissecting it, but at the same time not actually paying enough attention to what we eat.

What would happen if, for example, we were to start thinking about food as less of a commodity and more of a relationship?

Let me say straight off that I believe there is no such thing as healthy and unhealthy food. 'Wait!' I hear you cry. 'I bought this book because I want to be healthier and now she's telling me there is no such thing?' Let me add that of course there are foods that are 'better' for us from a nutritional standpoint and can improve our health, but it's simplistic to label one particular food good and another bad. We need to put it into context.

If I asked ten people, 'Which is healthier – a doughnut or an apple?' I would bet all my money (and I'm not a betting woman) that those ten people would say the apple. But how would it be if all you ate was apples? First, you would feel pretty sick, and second, you would likely be very malnourished from lack of calories and nutrients. So suddenly that apple isn't looking so healthy after all.

Calling a food 'healthy' assigns it value and isolates it from everything else we eat. What's wrong with that? Well, it doesn't reflect the way we actually eat. We don't eat specific nutrients – we eat foods in combinations and this dictates how our body processes and uses them. Unfortunately, we've developed a reductionist way of viewing foods, categorising them as good or bad. For example, butter = saturated fat = poor health. However, not many of us eat a knob of butter on its own, so spreading some on your toast in the morning as part of a nutritionally balanced diet is not going to do you any harm.

Perhaps the problem is that we are viewing our diet as a formula made of a specific amount of nutrients . . . x amount of carbohydrates + y amount of fat + z amount of protein +/- ∞ superfood(s) = health . . . when really, we get more from a varied diet than the sum of its parts.

Why do we look at food this way? I guess marketing is to blame, but science plays a part too. Since nutrients are invisible to the naked eye, it's up to scientists to tell producers what's in there and to producers to label the packaging with that information. When we browse grocery aisles we now see buzzwords – low fat, low calorie, healthy option, sugar free and superfood – printed prominently on the wrappings. The presence or absence of these labels decides which category the food should go in – healthy or unhealthy.

Apart from the simplistic nature of that approach, it can't predict how these foods will behave in the body because what happens in a lab doesn't always translate into real life. We all have different genes, different environments, and different social and cultural backgrounds. Humans are far more complicated than test tubes.

Now this is not to negate the science of food, and nutritional labelling is extremely important for certain individuals, such as high-performing athletes who need to consume specific amounts of carbohydrates and protein, or diabetics who need to be aware of how much sugar is in a specific food. That's why I've worked hard in my books to make this information accessible for those who need to know the finer details. However, the rest of us, who are not competing at elitist levels or do not have a medical requirement to follow a prescriptive diet, can have relatively flexible diets inclusive of all food groups, which will support our health.

Having discussed the importance of what we eat, I now want to look at the impact that how we eat has on our health.

MEDITERRANEAN DIET

Time and again, the one diet that is scientifically backed in terms of offering us the greatest health benefits and greatest longevity is the Mediterranean diet. This pattern of eating includes extra-virgin olive oil, fruit and vegetables, nuts and seeds, legumes and cereals, a moderate consumption of fish, poultry, dairy products and red wine, and a lower consumption of eggs, red and processed meats and processed foods. This diet focuses not on reducing individual nutrients, but on including a variety of good-quality, whole foods. It might sound too simple to be true, but the science is there to back it up. So are we who eat differently just over-complicating our dietary guidelines?

UNESCO (United Nations Educational, Scientific and Cultural Organisation) offers a very different, but refreshing, description of the Mediterranean diet as one that 'involves a set of skills, knowledge, rituals, symbols and traditions concerning crops, harvesting, fishing, animal husbandry, conservation, processing, cooking, and particularly the sharing and consumption of food'. It goes on to say that 'It plays a vital role in cultural spaces, festivals and celebrations, bringing together people of all ages, conditions and social classes.'

Which brings me to my next point: food is fuel . . . but it's so much more.

The Mediterranean diet is based on the traditional eating pattern of countries in southern Europe around the 1960s. The rates of chronic disease among those populations were among the lowest in the world and that continues to be the case today. However, their good bill of health is not simply due to the foods in their diet; it is also thanks to their relationship with food – how they eat it and who they eat it with.

In light of this, the Mediterranean diet food pyramid was recently revised to include cultural and lifestyle elements, such as cooking, physical activity, traditional, local and eco-friendly products, adequate rest, biodiversity and seasonality, and conviviality.

Maybe this is something that the rest of us are missing in our official guidelines? A true appreciation of food – from sourcing it, to cooking it, to sharing it.

Of course, lifestyles have changed massively since the 1960s, and not many families have the opportunity to enjoy dinner together every evening. Most of us work unsociable hours or have long commutes to work, which can mean leaving the house very early and getting home late, especially if we want to squeeze in a gym session or catch up with a friend for a drink after work. It's hard to slow down the pace of modern life, but we can make the most of the opportunities when we do have a little more time.

HOW TO USE THIS BOOK

To reflect the pattern of our busy lives, this book is split into two sections: FUEL UP and POWER DOWN.

THE FUEL UP SECTION is designed to suit the hectic days in your life when you need quick and easy recipes – portable breakfasts, fork-free lunches, energy-boosting snacks and batch-cook dinners – that will give you the fuel required to power through the working week without spending hours in the kitchen. This will help you to increase the time you have for unwinding after work and resting for the day ahead.

THE POWER DOWN SECTION is designed for the weekends, days off and holidays, when you have a little more time to enjoy and rediscover a love of food. I want you to be conscious not only of the type of food you eat, but also of how you cook and prepare it, how you eat it and who you share it with. In this section you will find lazy brunches, comforting family dinners, traditional breads, celebratory cakes and teatime treats.

Throughout the book you will find features on important topics, including nutrition, mindfulness and sleep. I want this book to be an all-round plan for healthy eating and living. I want it to help you forge a really healthy relationship with food; to embrace and enjoy eating healthy recipes with your family and friends; to enjoy exercise, reap the benefits of mindfulness and think about how to nourish yourself in every way.

For each recipe I've included a nutritional key. This is to make it easier for those with nutritional requirements and preferences to choose recipes suitable for their needs. This is not to highlight which recipes are healthier than others in any way and, as you delve deeper into the book, I hope you will understand that I believe all foods have a place in our diet to some extent. Remember, food is our only source of fuel and energy, but it is also there to be enjoyed.

Ve	VEGAN	**LOW GI**	LOW GI
V	VEGETARIAN	**MED GI**	MEDIUM GI
GF	GLUTEN FREE	**HIGH GI**	HIGH GI
LOW SUG	LOW SUGAR	**FIBRE XXg**	FIBRE CONTENT
LOW SALT	LOW SALT		

VEGAN: Plant-based recipes free of animal products.

VEGETARIAN: Recipes that do not contain animal meat or fish.

GLUTEN FREE: Recipes free of gluten-containing products.

LOW SUGAR: Recipes containing less than 5g of sugar per 100g.

LOW SALT: Recipes containing less than 0.3g of salt per 100g.

GI RATING: An approximate glycaemic index (GI) rating is listed under the nutrient information for each recipe, to indicate whether the dish produces a low, medium or high blood glucose response.

LOW GI: 55 or less
MEDIUM GI: 56–69
HIGH GI: 70+

FIBRE CONTENT: Estimated fibre content per serving. This is to help reach the target recommendation of 30g of fibre per day for adults.

Please note that the nutritional keys do not take into account any optional ingredients.

WHAT IS THE GLYCAEMIC INDEX?

The glycaemic index, or GI, is a ranking of how quickly different carbohydrates make your blood glucose levels rise after eating them. Food and drink with a high GI are digested quickly, causing a quick and sharp rise in blood glucose levels, which often drop just as rapidly, leaving us feeling sluggish. Low-GI foods and drink are digested more slowly, causing a steadier rise in blood glucose that typically keeps us feeling full for several hours after eating. These are sometimes referred to as 'slow-release' carbs. In general, high-GI foods are simple carbohydrates, such as sweets and dried fruit, and low-GI foods are usually complex carbohydrates, like oats, lentils and rye bread.

The glycaemic index can vary depending on a number of factors: the degree of ripeness, method of cooking and combination of different foods can all affect the GI of an individual food or ingredients within a recipe. Also, the GI doesn't take into account the fat or protein content, so a low GI value doesn't always represent a healthier or lower calorie food. Despite these shortcomings, when applied correctly the GI has been proven to be beneficial in health and athletic performance. In fact, if you have diabetes, it can be useful to understand the glycaemic index, as choosing foods with low-GI ratings can help control blood glucose. However, other factors must also be taken into account; it's also important to eat a balanced diet that features lots of fruits and vegetables, fibre, lean protein and healthy fats.

Many of the recipes in this book can be made suitable for vegetarians, vegans and those with gluten intolerance if certain basic ingredient swaps are made. In each case, do ensure the packaging specifies that the product is 100% gluten free, vegan or vegetarian.

INGREDIENT	GLUTEN-FREE (GF) REPLACEMENT	VEGAN REPLACEMENT
BAKING POWDER	Use certified 100% GF baking powder, e.g. Doves or Dr Oetker	–
BICARBONATE OF SODA	Use certified 100% GF bicarbonate of soda, e.g. Doves	–
BREADS/WRAPS	Use certified 100% GF bread/wraps	–
BUTTER	–	Coconut oil
BUTTERMILK	–	Combine 250ml coconut milk with 1 tbsp lemon juice and leave to stand for 5 minutes
CHEESE	–	Most popular cheeses (Cheddar, feta, Parmesan, etc.) have 100% vegan equivalents; try Nutcrafter Creamery, Vegusto, Violife and supermarket 'Free From' products
CHOCOLATE	–	Opt for dark chocolate only, including Cadbury's Bournville, Green & Black's, Moo Free and Plamil
CURRY PASTE	–	Some contain fish sauce or shrimp paste. Brands without include Blue Dragon, Maesri, Thai Taste
EGG	–	Flax egg (see tip, page 208) can be used in many bakes
FLOURS	Use 100% GF brands, such as Doves	–
HARISSA	Use 100% GF products, such as Mina or Harry Brand	–
HONEY	–	Maple syrup
MILK	–	Use plant-based alternatives, e.g. almond or soya milk
MISO	Use 100% GF brands, e.g. Clearspring	–
MUSTARD	Some products contain flour, so read the label and use GF brands, e.g. Duerr's	–
OATCAKES	Use 100% GF brands, e.g. Nairns	–
OATS	Use 100% GF brands, e.g. Mornflake	–
PASTA	Use 100% GF brands, e.g. Doves or supermarket 'Free From'	–
PESTO	–	Use a 'Free From' brand, e.g. Sacla, Zest
SOY SAUCE	Use 100% GF tamari, e.g. Clearspring, Kikkoman	–
STOCK	Use 100% GF brands, e.g. Kallo, Knorr	Use 100% dairy-free vegetable stock, e.g. Kallo, Knorr
TAHINI	Use 100% GF brands, e.g. Meridian, Raw Health	–
YOGURT		Use 100% GF brands, e.g. Meridian, Raw Health

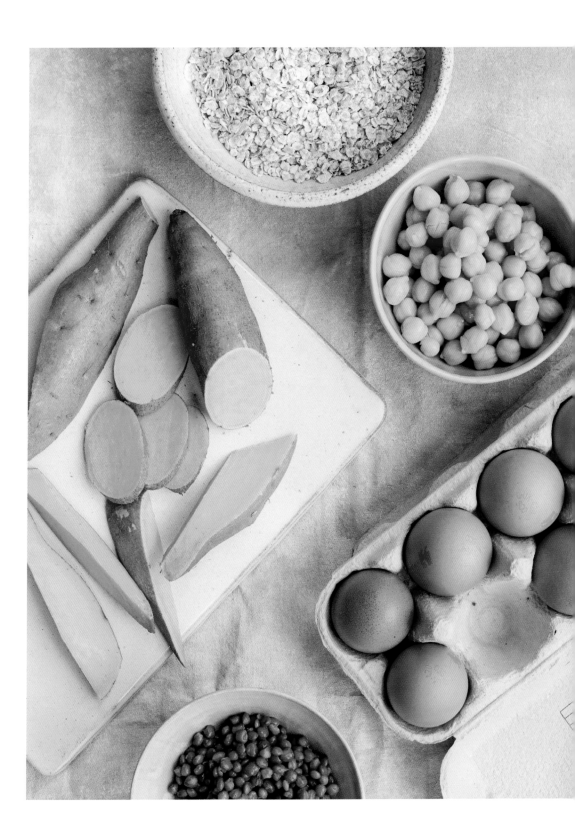

FIVE STORE-CUPBOARD SAVIOURS

I think most of us can relate to coming home from work after a long day, totally exhausted and absolutely ravenous. You get in and open up the fridge to find a lonely tub of butter, half a red pepper and zero inspiration. The energy and time required to cook a meal from scratch seems like too much effort, so you resort to a couple of slices of toast.

Here's the thing: no matter how great a cook you are, if there isn't food in the house and it's been a long day, you (and all of us) are way more likely to have a ready meal or order a take-away. No one wants to battle the evening rush hour, then drop into the supermarket, buy ingredients, go home and cook. But what's the solution? Having food in the house gives you a huge head start.

A well-stocked cupboard with some staple items that are versatile, nutritious and quick to cook is a life-saver. So I've picked out five of my favourites – chickpeas, sweet potatoes, lentils, eggs and oats – which I turn to over and again, especially when I'm tight on time and lacking inspiration, and show you at least ten different ways to cook with them. You can find these ingredients in any supermarket and they fit within anyone's budget.

1. CHICKPEAS

Typically, chickpeas can be bought tinned or dried. Find them beside the tinned beans and vegetables in nearly all supermarkets. Tinned chickpeas have already been cooked, so you only need to heat them up, or (if eating them cold) to drain and rinse them before use. Dried chickpeas need to be soaked overnight and simmered for 30-40 minutes before they can be eaten, but many argue that they taste better than tinned ones.

Chickpeas have a buttery texture and a slightly nutty taste, and are probably best known when combined with garlic and olive oil in a creamy dip called hummus. However, I've got a few more exciting ways you can eat them:

1. Chickpea, Carrot + Pepper Curry (page 96)
2. Spicy Prawn + Chickpea Stew (page 99)
3. Courgette + Harissa Falafels (page 91)
4. Carrot + Coriander Chickpea Burgers (page 86)
5. Sweet + Smoky Chickpea-stuffed Sweet Potatoes (page 202)
6. Peanut Butter + Chickpea Blondies (page 245)
7. The Italian One (page 67)
8. Baked Aubergine Hummus (page 130)
9. Chickpea Cookie Dough (page 149)
10. Sweet + Spicy Chickpea Croutons (page 148)

FACT: Chickpeas are an awesome source of plant protein, with roughly 8g per 100g serving.

2. SWEET POTATOES

Growing up, I don't remember coming across sweet potatoes very often. We always had Rooster, Kerr's Pink or Queens spuds. However, nowadays, sweet potatoes are almost easier to find than white potatoes – well, so it seems from Instagram!

But are sweet potatoes better for us than white potatoes or is it simply hype? In short, no. Both types contain vitamins and minerals, fibre and phytonutrients. Sweet potatoes, however, have an impressive amount of beta carotene, which is a precursor of vitamin A, with one standard serving offering the recommended daily intake.

Another argument for sweet potatoes is that they have a lower glycaemic index (GI) than white potatoes. However, the difference between the GI of a white potato and a sweet potato is also relatively small, so it is unlikely to make a massive difference.

So, side by side, they're both good guys and can both make up part of a healthy diet. However, it's a no-brainer that a bag of deep-fried potato crisps is not going to offer you the same nutritional benefits as a baked sweet potato. As with all fruits and vegetables, coloured potatoes and sweet potatoes are higher in phytonutrients, so keep your eyes peeled for purple spuds when you're next at a farm shop or market.

Here are ten great ways to enjoy sweet potatoes:

1. Sweet Potato Falafels (page 92)
2. Sweet Potato Fries (page 86)
3. Sweet Potato Toast (page 149)
4. Poached Eggs + Sweet Potato Fritters (page 156)
5. Sweet Potato, Hazelnut + Goat's Cheese Salad in a Pomegranate Dressing (page 100)
6. Mexican Loaded Sweet Potato Skins (page 196)
7. Sweet Potato Frittata (page 187)
8. Irish Sweet Potato Farls (page 174)
9. Spicy Sweet Potato + Peanut Butter Soup (page 77)
10. Sweet Potato Gratin (page 189)

3. LENTILS

Lentils are still relatively new to our diet in the UK and Ireland. They're a type of legume and come in many different shapes and colours. The most common ones you will find in the supermarket are green, red or black. They're high in protein, a great source of fibre, and also count towards one of your five-a-day. They are also incredibly cheap and very versatile to cook with. You can buy them dried, tinned or in microwaveable packets.

Here are some creative ways you can eat lentils:

1. Beetroot + Coconut Dhal (page 102)
2. Lentil Soup (page 74)
3. Lentil + Beetroot Burgers (page 84)
4. Smoky Sundried Tomato + Lentil Dip (page 131)
5. Lentil Shepherd's Pie (page 127)
6. Stuffed Peppers with Lentils + Feta (page 105)
7. Lentil + Kidney Bean Chilli (page 115)
8. The Middle Eastern One (page 68)
9. Bish-bash-bosh Chicken Tray Bake with Lentils + Roasted Vegetables (page 108)
10. Lentil Meatloaf (page 181)

> **FACT:** A 100g serving of cooked lentils contains approximately 10g of protein, about a quarter of our daily requirement.

4. OATS

Ah, oats. My favourite grain. Before going to school when I was little, I always had a bowl of porridge topped with a spoonful of jam or honey. I still love it now, and not only for breakfast, but as part of my lunch, dinner and snacks.

Oats are a great source of fibre, particularly a soluble fibre called beta-glucan, which has been proven to reduce cholesterol. Just 3g of beta-glucan per day appears to be the optimal amount to achieve this in both people with normal and high cholesterol. A 40g serving of porridge contains 2g of beta-glucan, so your morning oats and a couple of homemade oatcakes should get you to your daily target. Opt for jumbo oats or steel-cut oats, which are slower to digest and therefore less likely to give you the rapid sugar hit of instant oats.

Here are a few different ways of including oats in your diet:

1. Porridge, sweet or savoury (pages 36, 38)
2. Toasted Oat, Quinoa + Stewed Apple Yogurt Pot (page 52)
3. Chocolate Orange Granola (page 47)
4. Oatcakes (page 215)
5. Oat Goujons + Homemade Ketchup (page 178)

6. Cranberry + Pecan Granola Bars, Fig Roll Oat Bars or Trail Mix Bars (pages 62, 134, 138)
7. Pistachio, Apple + Raspberry Bircher Muesli (page 35)
8. Porridge Bread (page 208)
9. Rhubarb Crumble (page 221)
10. Chocolate Chip Oatmeal Cookies (page 145)

5. EGGS

High in protein, vitamins A, D and B12, eggs are great to include in the diet from a nutritional point of view – but what about the cholesterol, I hear you say?

For years scientists and doctors believed that eggs and dietary cholesterol caused high blood cholesterol and, therefore, increased the risk of heart disease and stroke. However, as more research has been carried out over the years with better scientific techniques, the evidence appears to show that dietary cholesterol does not necessarily translate to high blood cholesterol! We don't have a recommended daily allowance of eggs in our guidelines and the question as to how many eggs are too many is a very difficult one to ask without any context. Eggs are also a source of saturated fat, which may increase our risk of cardiovascular disease if eaten to excess. As with anything in life, everything in moderation!

Here are ten great ways of enjoying eggs in a varied diet:

1. Smoked Salmon-wrapped Asparagus with Poached Eggs + Tomatoes (page 154)
2. Dressed-up Tomato + Cheese Omelette (page 59)
3. Sweet Potato Frittata (page 187)
4. Dippy Eggs + Root Vegetable Soldiers (page 159)
5. The Food Medic Fry-up (page 160)
6. Scrambled Egg, Red Pepper + Cream Cheese Pitta Pocket (page 56)
7. Shakshuka Eggs + Crumbled Feta (page 162)
8. French Toast with Berry Compote (page 173)
9. Spelt + Buckwheat Pancakes or Chocolate Chip Banana Pancakes (pages 168, 171)
10. The French One (page 66)

STORE-CUPBOARD ESSENTIALS

This is my list of store-cupboard staples that I always have in the house. It may seem like a lot but they have a long shelf-life and often come in large quantities that you can use over and over again. I'm not including the ingredients that I would use on a one-off basis or fresh and frozen ingredients. This is simply to help you build a good pantry full of basic ingredients that you will get the most use out of. Of course, this is not a definitive list but I hope it will give you some ideas and inspiration. As with all of the ingredients in this book, you should be able to pick up most of them in any supermarket!

BAKING	Almond extract, Baking powder, Bicarbonate of soda, Black molasses, Cocoa powder, Cornflour, Flours (buckwheat, rye, spelt, regular wheat or gluten-free plain flour), Ground almonds, Vanilla extract
DRIED FRUIT + SUGARS	Apricots, Dates, Figs, Raisins, Brown sugar, Coconut sugar, Honey, Maple syrup
GRAINS + STARCHY VEGETABLES	Butternut squash, Couscous, Oats, Pasta, Quinoa, Rice, Sweet potatoes, White potatoes
LEGUMES + TINNED VEGETABLES	Black beans, Butter beans, Chickpeas, Lentils, Red kidney beans, Tinned chopped tomatoes, Tinned plum tomatoes, Tinned sweetcorn
NUTS + SEEDS	Almonds, Cashews, Hazelnuts, Peanuts, Pistachios, Walnuts, Chia seeds, Pumpkin seeds, Sesame seeds, Sunflower seeds, Flaxseed/linseed, Nut butter, Tahini
OILS + BUTTER	Avocado oil, Coconut oil, Grass-fed butter, Extra-virgin olive oil, Rapeseed oil, Toasted sesame oil
SAUCES, CONDIMENTS + VINEGARS	Coconut milk, Harissa paste, Hot chilli sauce, Mirin, Miso paste, Mustard (Dijon and wholegrain), Tamari sauce or soy sauce, Thai curry paste (red or green), Tomato purée, Vinegar (apple cider, balsamic, white wine)
SPICES, HERBS + SEASONING	Chilli powder, Chilli flakes, Cloves (whole), Dried basil, Dried garlic, Dried mixed herbs, Dried oregano, Dried parsley, Dried rosemary, Dried thyme, Garam masala, Ground cinnamon, Ground ginger, Ground turmeric, Ground nutmeg, Ground cumin, Ground coriander, Paprika (smoked), Pepper, black, Salt, Stock cubes

IS COCONUT OIL A SUPERFOOD OR SUPERVILLAIN?

Claims that coconut oil is 'as unhealthy as beef fat and butter' made headlines in 2017 after the American Heart Association (AHA) released a review of the data on the effects of dietary saturated fat intake on cardiovascular disease (see page 43 for more information). Coconut oil is certainly not a superfood (it never has been) but it probably isn't a supervillain either. Use it sparingly in cooking, as you would with butter or any other fat, but make use of other oils also. I will still be using coconut oil in certain dishes, particularly in my desserts and Asian recipes, but I also use a variety of other oils in my cooking, such as olive oil, sesame seed oil, avocado oil and butter.

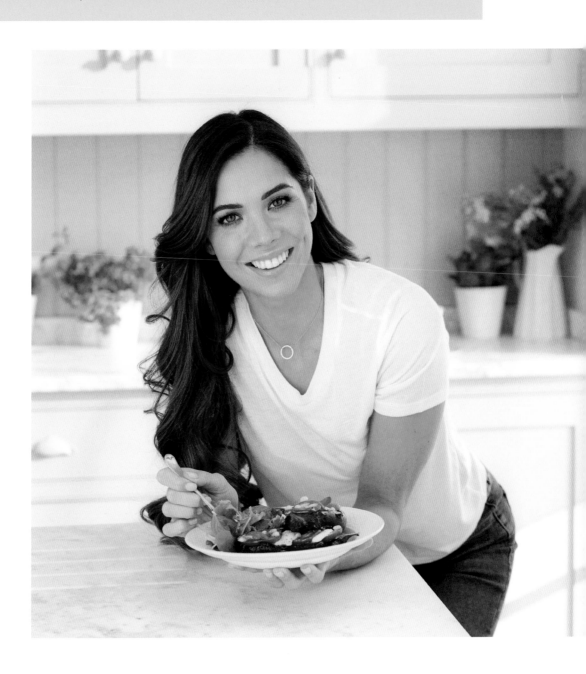

USEFUL EQUIPMENT

I'm a very simple woman. I don't like clutter and I don't buy things that I don't need, so I am not massively into gadgets or gizmos for the kitchen. However, there are a few essentials that I use almost daily and I think you too will find them useful when using this book.

AIRTIGHT CONTAINERS AND CLIP-TOP JARS: In my kitchen I have containers in every shape and size – little ones for carrying nuts and fruit, medium ones for lunches and dinner, and larger ones for storing batches of soup, stew and curry in the fridge or freezer. I use large clip-top jars for my salads and homemade pickles, and smaller ones for transporting my overnight oats and storing homemade jams. I also save peanut butter jars (glass ones) and use them for oats or DIY yogurt pots (see pages 52–55). And don't forget to add a label and date to your containers; you can get lovely chalkboard stickers that can be wiped clean and reused time after time.

FOOD PROCESSOR: At university I bought the most budget-friendly food processor I could find (less than £20) and tried to make nut butter. It was working so hard that it almost went up in flames. It choked the next day. RIP. I learnt my lesson, and invested in a sturdy food processor with various attachments for doing lots different tasks. I'm happy to tell you that it's still alive and kicking.

GOOD KNIVES: I only fully appreciated the benefits of good knives when I really got into cooking. Not only do they make you feel super-sleek when slicing and chopping, but you won't have to fight to get the blade out of a dense sweet potato or butternut squash.

HAND BLENDER: When I was growing up, my mum did most things by hand as she had very few kitchen gadgets. But one thing she often used was a hand blender (and a hostess trolley, which she will tell you is the best thing since sliced bread if you ever get a minute with her). She made a lot of soup for us as kids so that we'd have something warm and nourishing on getting home from school, and to keep us going until dinner later on in the evening. The hand blender ensured the soup was chunk-free so that we couldn't pick out the vegetables we didn't like. (Mum 1 – Kids 0.) These days I also use my hand blender for making creamy dips, mashes, sauces and smoothies.

KITCHEN SCALES AND MEASURING JUGS: I find kitchen scales really useful, particularly when it comes to baking, but also when weighing meat and grains. For accurate liquid measurement, I also think you need a clearly marked jug.

STURDY PICNIC CUTLERY: How many forks have you taken to work never to see them again? Or how many random pieces of cutlery do you have in your house that you've taken from work and forgotten to return? Too many, I suspect. I suggest you invest in a good set of picnic cutlery and use it solely for your meals-on-the-go. Browse online to find foldable plastic spoons, knives and forks, or buy a packet of wooden utensils, which can be washed and reused countless times and are cheap enough to lose without counting the cost.

VEGETABLE PEELER: I may be the only health blogger who doesn't own a spiraliser, and although I have nothing against spiralised vegetables (it does look pretty cool), I wouldn't call it an essential item to have in your kitchen. I think a vegetable peeler is a cheaper and less fussy alternative, which makes equally good ribbons from carrots, courgettes and cucumbers (great in salads and stir-fries). For even finer ribbons you can use a julienne peeler, which looks like a vegetable peeler with a deeply serrated blade.

ZIPLOCK BAGS: I'm trying to reduce my plastic consumption, but if you're short of fridge or freezer space, ziplock bags are a great way to store batch-cooked meals. They can also be washed and reused.

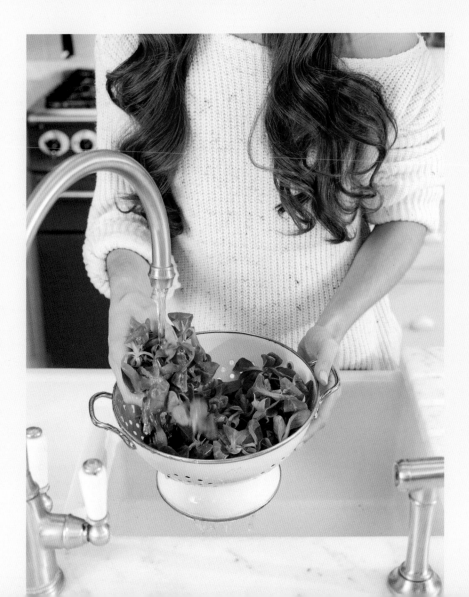

FUEL UP

Our biggest obstacle when it comes to cooking and eating well is time. After a busy day at work, no one (myself included) has the time, energy or motivation to spend hours in the kitchen. Although I would love to spend more time experimenting with fancy ingredients and cooking up something new every evening, that is simply not feasible. My busy schedule as a doctor means that I have no choice but to be extremely time-efficient and organised about food, so I prep things in advance. I can knock up a week of lunches and a few dinners pretty easily, but that was not always the case.

It's such a lovely feeling to be on the way home after a busy day and know that a lovely dinner is waiting. So I'm going to share with you my insider tips on how to be a dab hand at meal prep.

MEAL PREP HACKS

Here are a few key things that will help you to save time and stay on track with healthy eating.

WRITE A SHOPPING LIST

How many times have you walked into a supermarket to pick up milk and walked out with a basket full of random items that you didn't really need and will probably never use, and you've gone and forgotten the milk? I put my hand up and say I am so guilty of this.

Well, call me old-school, but I love a good shopping list. It's really satisfying to tick things off – so much so that I will often add a completed task to the list just so I can cross it off . . . is it just me, or do you do that too?

In addition to that feeling of pride you get when you've worked your way through a list, it's a total life-saver for many other reasons:

- You're less likely to forget the things you need.

- It saves you time wandering the aisles shooting in the dark by aimlessly tossing things into your trolley: 'I think I need eggs.' 'Do I need eggs?' 'I'd better buy some eggs, or did I buy them yesterday?'

- It helps you to meal-plan for the week, so you have less of a ready-steady-cook situation with a courgette and a tin of tuna when you get in from work.

- It reduces food waste. If you're not realistically going to use a fresh food item that week, don't buy it.

- It helps you save money because you're less like to impulse-buy that odd-shaped vegetable that you've no idea how to cook or eat.

- It will stop you 'eating with your eyes'. I'm sure you can relate to this when you go shopping on an empty stomach and suddenly you're the proud owner of aisle six.

If you're stuck for inspiration on your shopping list, take a look at my store-cupboard essentials (see page 20), which includes all the dried and tinned foods that I turn to time again. Keep in mind that my list is just a guide, not something definitive. Scribble down some notes, add your favourites, and be inspired to try something new. In addition to the usual items on my shopping list, I also like to buy a vegetable that I have never cooked with or haven't eaten in some time. I call it my vegetable of the week.

TAKE SHORT CUTS

As a rule, when people consult me about improving their health, I advise them to cut down on the amount of processed food they buy. Obviously, most foods we consume have undergone some form of processing, so it's unrealistic to cut them out completely, but there is a huge difference between a pot of noodles in a powdered 'sauce' and a packet of pre-chopped carrot batons. So you need to use your own judgement a little here – sometimes the processed or packaged version is just as good an option as its raw predecessor when we are running short on time.

Some of my favourite time-saving foods include:

- Frozen fruit and vegetables

- Microwaveable packets of grains and pulses (e.g. lentils)

- Ready-cooked chicken, salmon fillets and smoked fish

- Vegetable and chicken stock

- Cartons and tins of beans

- Carrot batons and other chopped vegetables (it seems lazy, I know, but sometimes having them pre-chopped is a godsend and encourages me to eat more vegetables as a result)

- Hummus (although I have a super-easy recipe on page 130)

- Nut butter (choose one with as few extra ingredients as possible – all you need in there is nuts)

- Dried herbs (see page 20)

- Rye and sourdough bread (I love making my own, but I totally understand that sometimes you just want the damn stuff without faffing around)

BEFRIEND THE FREEZER

Whether you're cooking for one person or six, preparing meals in advance and freezing them will help you to cut down on waste and save time midweek. Among the recipes in this book you will find lots that are suitable for batch-cooking and can be portioned out for the week, or frozen for times when you're too busy to cook or plan ahead. My mum taught me how to make full use of my freezer, and it's saved me a lot of time and money over the years.

Maximise freezer space by storing stuff in ziplock bags rather than boxes, and stack them on top of one another like a pile of pillows. Grab some tape and label them with a black marker so you don't mix up your veggie chilli with your bolognese sauce. Also, don't forget to include the date of freezing. (We all have some items from the dark ages lurking in the back of the freezer, but nothing lasts forever. If you're unsure how long something has been in there, I suggest you throw it out.)

Portion up before freezing. Most of us buy our meat in bulk because it's much cheaper than buying an individual portion. However, freezing in bulk, means defrosting in bulk, which often means you have to cook more than you need and you end up wasting leftovers – not such a money-saver after all. Separating food into portions before putting in the freezer makes it much easier to

defrost the amount you need, and also means you don't have to wait ages for a huge block of chicken breasts to defrost. Similarly, divide batch-meals into individual portions before freezing them. All you have to do is whip out one bagful and place it in the microwave for a super-quick dinner or lunch.

Freeze the unusual. Here are some foods that you might not have considered freezing, but doing so will change your life.

- Slice a loaf before freezing it. In the morning you can simply separate a couple of slices and pop them in the toaster on the defrost and toast settings. Say goodbye to mouldy bread for good.

- Freeze fresh herbs and simply crumble them into dishes whenever you need to. Go a step further and freeze chopped mint with some water in an ice-cube tray to add to cold drinks and cocktails.

- Frozen bananas (see tip, page 48) make the creamiest smoothies, and blended on their own make a one-ingredient ice cream. Freezing them also means that those spotty specimens in your fruit bowl don't need to go to waste.

- Make and freeze the tomato sauce on page 120 and defrost as needed for a super-speedy pasta dish.

- Add a teaspoon of peanut butter to the middle of a pitted date and freeze for an instant toffee treat when those sugar cravings hit.

PACKED LUNCH RENAISSANCE

It's time to make the packed lunch cool again, so here are a few ideas for doing just that:

LUNCH-SHARE. Just as work colleagues car-share, how about lunch-sharing with a work friend? Take turns making lunch on alternate weeks or alternate days to halve the time and effort involved and to keep things interesting. You could do this with your housemate or partner, or even your mum.

DOUBLE UP ON DINNER PORTIONS. When preparing dinner, make twice the amount, saving half to eat on another day. Pop it in an open plastic container, allow to cool, then seal and refrigerate until needed. Simple. This is an easy way to prep a meal in advance without getting into a mammoth late-night cooking session and its cleaning aftermath.

PACK IT PROPERLY. One of my greatest paranoias is a leaky lunchbox. At uni, I used to buy cheap plastic boxes in pound stores, but they never had the best-quality seal, which meant smelly salad juice at the bottom of my bag for days. Spend some time and a bit more cash investing in some lunchboxes that you won't need to replace by the end of the month. You can now buy really good bento boxes with different compartments, or old-fashioned stainless steel boxes, or do what I do and layer it all inside a clip-top jar (which looks much fancier than it actually is and you will feel super-smug whipping it out in the office).

PACK A SURPRISE. If you're packing lunch for someone else in the house, it's a really lovely idea to leave something in their lunchbox to surprise them. This can be as simple as a little note on paper, a message inked onto the skin of a banana, something funny drawn on a hard-boiled egg, or even a flower . . . Who said romance was dead?

SCHOOL LUNCHBOX TIPS

- Ask your children what they would like for lunch, or offer them some healthy options to choose from. It's likely they will be more inclined to eat what they've chosen or had a part in choosing.

- Take them shopping and let them have a say (to a certain extent) in what goes in the trolley. Maybe ask them to pick out a fruit and vegetable they want to try that week. At the end of the day, you want to send your kids to school with food you know they'll eat and enjoy, but it's also worth including an additional new fruit or veg for them to try, without getting stressed if they don't eat it. Taste preferences develop over time.

- Let them help you to prepare lunch the night before by filling up their water bottle or choosing a piece of fruit. PS If they want fruit juice, the recommended daily serving is 150ml, so water it down to make it go a little further.

- Do some baking with them at the weekend for healthy snacks throughout the week.

- Give them a reason to be excited for lunch by using cookie cutters to make shapes out of bread, cheese and fruit, or draw something on the skin of their banana or orange.

- Chop fruit into bite-sized pieces so that it's easier to eat, adding a squeeze of lemon juice to stop it going brown.

- Add a portion of fork-free veggies, such as cherry tomatoes and carrot sticks, and a little tub of homemade dip (see pages 130–131).

BREAKFAST ON THE GO

I'll admit there are some mornings when the best we can do is tear ourselves from under the duvet, grab a fistful of cereal and dash out the door. A home-cooked breakfast is not a realistic expectation during a busy working week, but that doesn't mean we need to go hungry or settle for a sugary breakfast bar to fill the gap until lunchtime. You would be surprised how many nutritious breakfast ideas require very little effort to put into practice.

In this chapter, I'm going to open your mind to an array of grab-and-go breakfasts, from super-easy Carrot + Apple Breakfast Muffins (see page 60), which you can make ahead of time to nibble on the train, to gourmet yogurt pots that you can quickly assemble in the morning, and fast-blast smoothies that you can sip on while walking to work.

OVERNIGHT OATS FOUR WAYS

Overnight oats are essentially a no-cook method of making porridge. As the name suggests, you make them ahead and leave them in the fridge overnight, ready to grab and go in the morning. You can make them in a plastic box or clip-top jar, but . . . insider tip coming up! . . . I like to use empty peanut butter jars to carry mine, especially when there's a little bit of peanut butter left inside. Not only are these pots delicious, but they are packed full of fibre from the oats, boosted with protein from yogurt, and offer a good source of omega 3 fatty acids from chia and flaxseed.

BASIC OVERNIGHT OATS

SERVES 1

This is my base recipe, which you can jazz up and make your own.

40g oats
100g natural Greek yogurt
120ml milk
1 tbsp chia seeds or
 ground flaxseed
½ tsp vanilla extract
1 tbsp maple syrup
 or honey

Put all the ingredients into a small mixing bowl and whisk together. Spoon into a jar and seal tightly. Refrigerate overnight, or for at least 4 hours.

CHOCO-PEANUT OVERNIGHT OATS

SERVES 1

Basic Overnight Oats
 ingredients (see above)
1 tbsp peanut butter,
 plus extra serving
1 tbsp cocoa powder
1 tbsp peanuts, chopped

Put all the ingredients, except the peanuts, into a small mixing bowl and whisk together. Spoon into a jar and seal tightly. Refrigerate overnight, or for at least 4 hours.

Sprinkle the chopped peanuts on top and dot with extra peanut butter before serving.

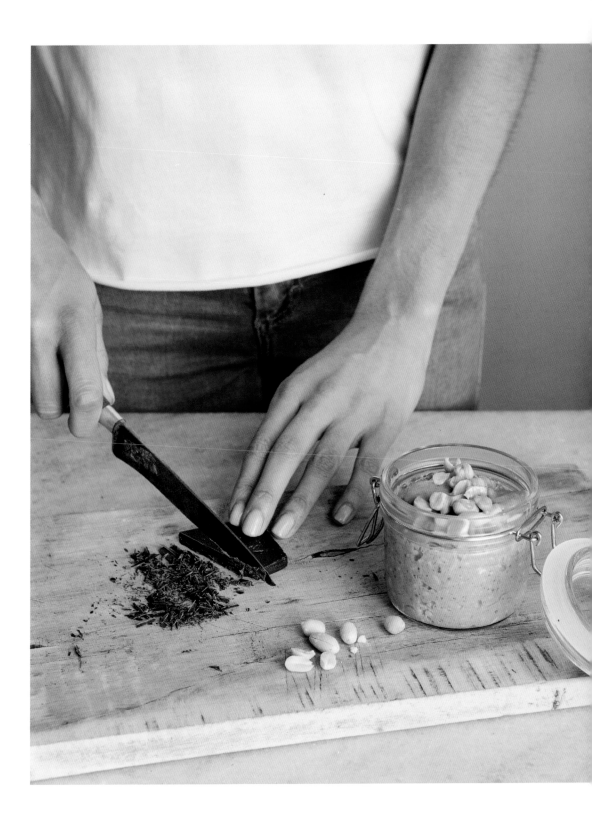

CARROT, PECAN + RAISIN OVERNIGHT OATS

SERVES 1

Basic Overnight Oats
  ingredients (see page 30)
½ carrot, finely grated
½ tsp ground cinnamon,
  plus extra to sprinkle
½ tsp ground nutmeg
2 tbsp raisins
2 tbsp pecans, chopped

Put all the ingredients, except the pecans, into a small mixing bowl and whisk together. Spoon into a jar and seal tightly. Refrigerate overnight, or for at least 4 hours.

Sprinkle the chopped pecans and some extra cinnamon on top before eating.

BLUEBERRY + CINNAMON OVERNIGHT OATS

SERVES 1

Basic Overnight Oats
  ingredients (see page 30)
½ tsp ground cinnamon
Handful of blueberries,
  plus extra to sprinkle

Put all the ingredients, except the blueberries, into a small mixing bowl and whisk together. Stir in the blueberries, spoon the mixture into a jar and seal tightly. Refrigerate overnight, or for at least 4 hours.

Sprinkle the extra blueberries on top before eating.

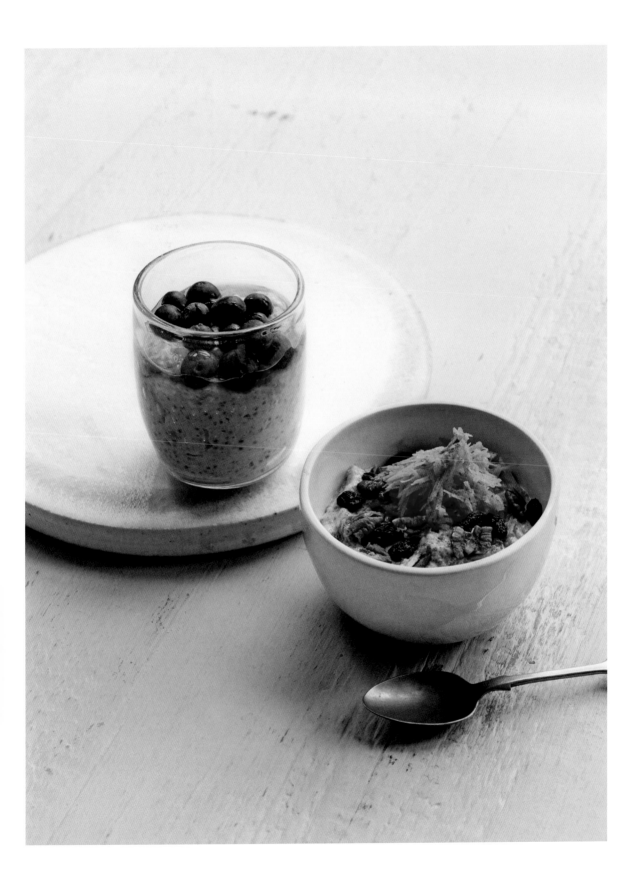

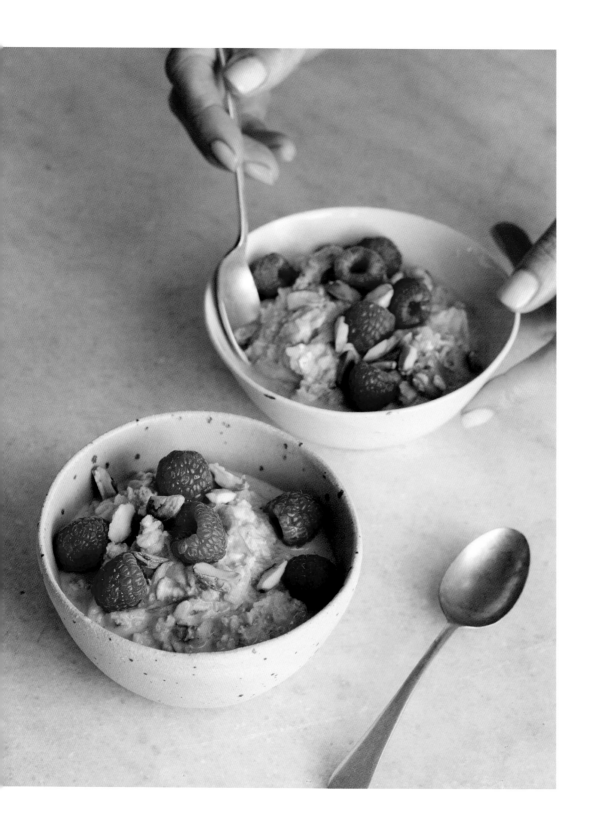

PISTACHIO, APPLE + RASPBERRY BIRCHER MUESLI

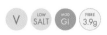

SERVES 2

This is the perfect recipe for the spring and summer months when it's too warm for porridge but you still want something delicious and filling for breakfast. It's also perfect for anyone who feels that they don't have time for breakfast in the morning because prepping this the night before takes that obstacle out of the equation. As this recipe serves two, how about treating your other half to something special before work?

50g oats

½ tsp ground cinnamon

½ tsp vanilla extract

1 apple, grated

1 tbsp honey or maple syrup

200ml milk

2 tbsp natural yogurt

Handful of raspberries, plus extra to sprinkle

25g pistachios, chopped

Combine the oats, cinnamon, vanilla, apple, honey and milk in a bowl. Cover and leave to soak overnight, or for at least 2 hours.

Stir in the yogurt and raspberries, then divide the mixture between 2 bowls or jars.

Sprinkle the extra raspberries and the pistachios over each serving before eating.

PORRIDGE WITH CARAMELISED APPLE + ALMOND BUTTER

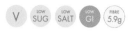

SERVES 2

It's no secret that I love porridge, and it's certainly no secret that I love nut butter. I almost broke out in a cold sweat when I thought I had forgotten to include a porridge recipe in this book. Let's be real – porridge can be pretty boring on its own. It's all about the toppings, and I've chosen my favourite to share with you.

1 tbsp butter

1 tbsp maple syrup

½ tsp ground cinnamon

½ tsp ground nutmeg

1 apple, cored and chopped into chunks

80g oats

440ml milk or water

Salt

2 tbsp almond butter, to serve

Melt the butter in a small pan over a medium heat. Stir in the maple syrup, cinnamon and nutmeg, then add the apple, stirring until fully coated. Cook for 5–7 minutes, until the apples have softened.

Place the oats and milk in a small saucepan and add a pinch of salt. Bring to the boil and simmer for 4–5 minutes, until all the liquid is absorbed, stirring from time to time and watching carefully that the mixture doesn't stick to the bottom of the pan. (This step can be done in the microwave to save time – 2–3 minutes on full power.)

Serve the porridge topped with the caramelised apple and dotted with the almond butter.

VARIATION: *For a nut-free version, omit the nuts, or combine 1 tablespoon tahini with 1 tablespoon maple syrup for a quick salted caramel drizzle.*

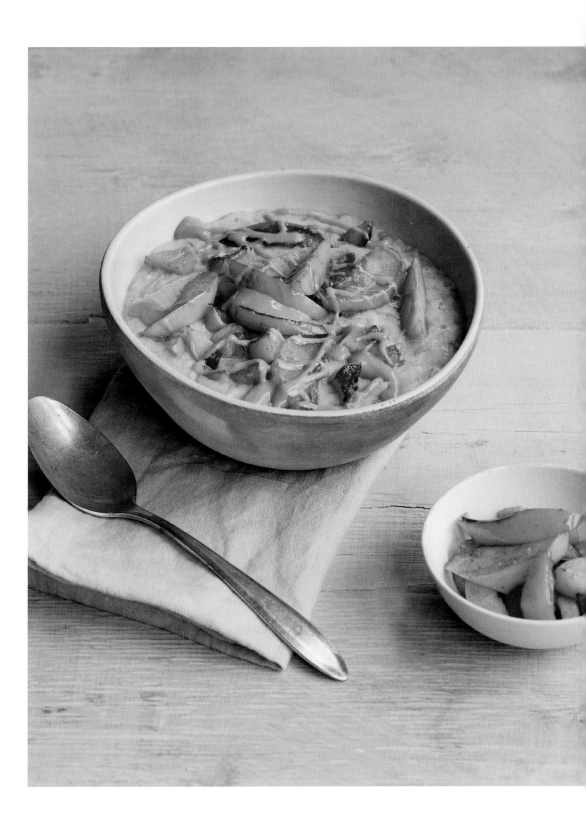

SAVOURY COURGETTE, PESTO + SUNDRIED TOMATO PORRIDGE

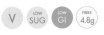

SERVES 1

When I first tried this recipe, I got in the door at 4pm, after a day of meetings, and I had yet to have lunch. As you can imagine, I was ravenous, but my fridge was virtually empty. I had to think fast. I had eggs, milk and some leftover vegetables, and in my cupboard I had some oats, so I wondered whether to make an omelette or porridge. Then it came to me: why not do both? So I whipped up this quick little meal and hesitantly tested the final product. It was amazing! Savoury porridge may be unfamiliar to you, but please don't knock it until you try it. It's basically like risotto, minus the faff.

You could obviously prepare savoury oats a thousand different ways by stirring in different ingredients and flavourings. I love that it's an easy vehicle for getting in lots of nutrients and fibre, not to mention the protein and healthy fats from the egg.

40g oats

½ courgette (about 50g), grated

175–200ml milk or water

¼ tsp salt

¼ tsp dried basil

¼ tsp dried oregano

1 tbsp pesto

1 tbsp grated Parmesan cheese

2–3 sundried tomatoes, chopped

½ tbsp oil

1 free-range egg

1 tbsp pine nuts

2–3 fresh basil leaves, torn

Salt and black pepper

Put the oats, courgette, milk, salt and herbs in a saucepan over medium heat and cook gently for 3–5 minutes, stirring occasionally until the mixture is thick and creamy.

Stir in the pesto, Parmesan and tomatoes. Keep warm over a very low heat.

Heat the oil in a frying pan, then fry the egg until cooked to your liking.

Spoon the oats into a bowl and top with the egg, pine nuts and torn basil leaves.

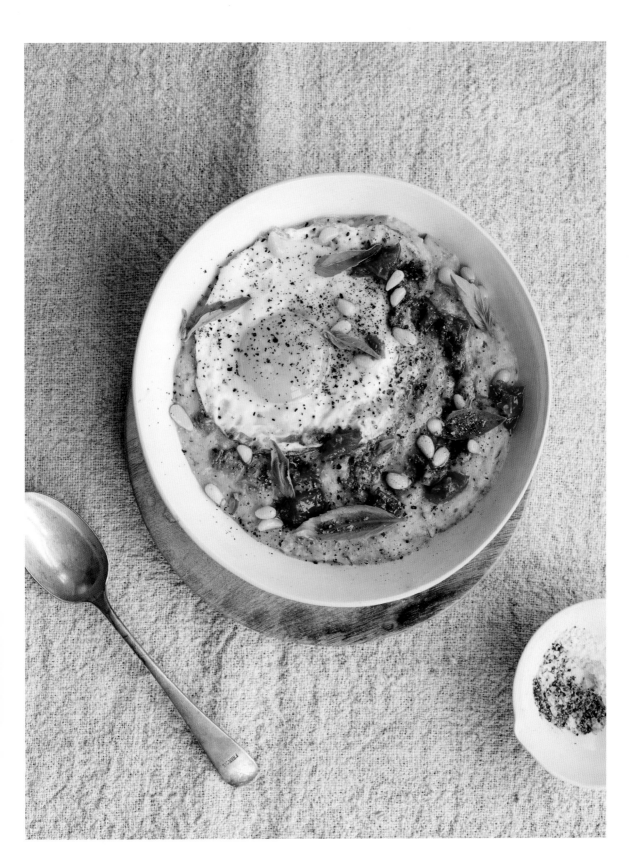

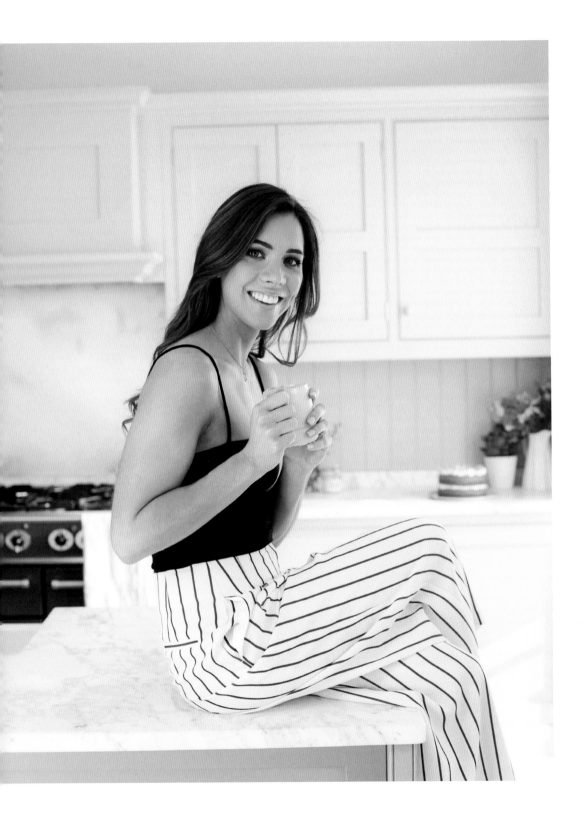

MACRONUTRIENTS

Macro means 'large', so in the context of nutrition, macronutrients are those foods that the human body needs in large amounts, namely protein, fats and carbohydrates.

PROTEIN

What does it do?

Protein is used to build and repair muscles, cartilage, ligaments, skin, hair and lots of other tissues, as well as making important enzymes, hormones and antibodies (defence cells) for our immune system.

What types are there?

- Proteins are made up of single units called amino acids.

- There are approximately 20 amino acids, some of which are essential, meaning that they must come from our diet as we can't make them ourselves.

- Dietary proteins that have all the essential amino acids are called 'complete' proteins, and this includes mostly animal foods, such as meat, fish, eggs and dairy products, and a handful of plant foods, such as quinoa, hemp protein and chia seeds.

- Proteins that contain some, but not all, of the essential amino acids are called 'incomplete' proteins. Examples include vegetables, grains, nuts and legumes.

How much do you need?

A moderately active adult should have 0.75g protein per kilogram of bodyweight.

People who are active require more protein, and the amount varies from 1.2 to 2g, depending on the type, intensity and duration of exercise. For example, those who do strength training (e.g. weight lifting) require more than those who do endurance training (e.g. running).

What does a serving look like?

- 1 fillet of fish (try to eat 2 portions of oily fish, such as salmon or mackerel, a week)

- 1 chicken breast or palm-sized piece of steak

- 125g cooked pulses (drained weight), such as chickpeas or lentils

- 1 small tub of dairy or soya yogurt (plant-based yogurts tend to be low in protein)

- 2 free-range eggs

- 600ml semi-skimmed milk

IS EATING MORE PROTEIN BETTER FOR YOU?

Some bodybuilders consume huge amounts of protein, up to 3g per kilo of bodyweight per day. However, there is no evidence that consuming more protein than you need will lead to further (or faster) muscle or strength gains. Sorry, boys.

FATS

What do they do?

Fat is essential for the absorption of fat-soluble vitamins (A, D, E, K), it provides us with energy, keeps us warm, sustains a healthy brain and nervous system, and even keeps our hair glossy and our skin glowing.

What types are there?

There are three main types of dietary fat: saturated fats, unsaturated fats and trans fats.

UNSATURATED FATS: There are two types – monounsaturated and polyunsaturated fatty acids.

Monounsaturated fats (MUFAs) are found in olive oil and nut oils, avocados, nuts and seeds. A diet high in monounsaturated fats is associated with improved cholesterol levels and an overall reduced risk of heart disease.

Polyunsaturated fats (PUFAs), mainly in the form of omega 3 and omega 6, are essential to our diet because the body cannot make them itself. Omega 3 is anti-inflammatory and has not only been associated with a reduction in the risk of heart disease and stroke, but also appears to have a role in brain performance and the prevention of mental health disorders, such as depression, and cognitive disorders, such as dementia.

- Omega 6 is found in vegetable oils.

- Omega 3 is found in oily fish (salmon, mackerel and tuna), flaxseeds and walnuts, and omega 3 supplements.

SATURATED FATS: These tend to be solid at room temperature – think butter, coconut oil and the marbling in beef. (See box on opposite page for further information.)

TRANS FATS: These occur naturally in small amounts in some animal foods, such as meat and dairy products, but most of the trans fatty acids in the diet are created by artificially hardening unsaturated fats (e.g. vegetable oils) through a process called hydrogenation. Trans fats are found in hard margarines, 'partially hydrogenated' oils, baked goods such as biscuits and cakes, fried foods and many other processed foods.

There is a broad scientific consensus that a high intake of trans fats significantly increases the risk of heart disease, and may also be associated with increased risk of other cardiovascular diseases, obesity and type 2 diabetes.

How much do you need?

Total fat intake should be about 35% or less, with only 11% of this coming from saturated fat. Instead of focusing on numbers/percentages, a good place to start would be focusing on getting most of your fat intake from the best sources – the foods high in monounsaturated and polyunsaturated fats.

Intake of trans fatty acids should not exceed 2% of food energy. In the UK we are consuming only 0.5–0.6% of our calories as trans fats, so we are well within recommended maximum levels.

What does a serving look like?

- ½ avocado
- 1 tablespoon olive oil
- 1 tablespoon nut butter or tahini
- 1 tablespoon seeds
- 1 thumb-sized piece of cheese
- 2 tablespoons nuts
- 1 portion oily fish (salmon, sardines, tuna, mackerel)

CARBOHYDRATES

What do they do?

Carbohydrate, in the form of glucose, is the main source of energy in the body, fuelling all our activities, from simply breathing to running a marathon. Any glucose that we don't need to use immediately for energy can be converted to its storage form, glycogen, and stored in the liver and muscles. We can convert glycogen back to glucose if we need it, such as when we need additional fuel during exercise.

What types are there?

Carbohydrates can be split into two broad groups, simple and complex, depending on their structure, which dictates how the body handles them. A third group is dietary fibre.

SIMPLE CARBOHYDRATES include sugars, such as glucose, fructose, sucrose and lactose. They are made up either of one sugar unit (monosaccharide) or two sugar units (disaccharides). Due to their simple structure, they are very quickly absorbed into the bloodstream, giving us a quick supply of energy. This isn't necessarily a bad thing, though. Simple carbohydrates are found in dairy products, which offer us important vitamins and minerals, such as calcium and vitamin D, and are also in fruits and vegetables, which are full of vitamins and minerals, phytochemicals (more on this later) and fibre. However, simple carbohydrates are also found in refined grains (white bread, white rice and pasta), sweets and cakes, and sugary drinks. Although these foods provide us with energy (and pleasure), they don't provide us with many nutrients, so we should eat them as little as possible in our diet.

COMPLEX CARBOHYDRATES are largely found in whole grains, starchy vegetables, legumes, nuts and seeds. They are made up of long chains of sugar units, known as polysaccharides. Their complex structure means they are broken down more slowly than simple sugars, and therefore provide energy over a longer period of time. This causes less of a dramatic spike in our blood glucose and subsequent insulin response. The high fibre is also very satisfying, keeping us feeling full for longer.

Dietary fibre, also known as roughage (at least by my mum), is the non-digestible part of plants in our diet. Unlike other carbohydrates, it doesn't provide us with much energy, but it helps to keep the gut healthy by encouraging smooth transit of digested food through the bowel and by nourishing healthy gut bacteria. A diet high in fibre is also associated with a lower risk of heart disease, stroke, type 2 diabetes and bowel cancer.

There are two types of fibre – soluble and insoluble.

SOLUBLE FIBRE is found in grains such as oats and rye, fruits such as figs and prunes, legumes such as peas and chickpeas, and vegetables such as carrots and potatoes. This type of fibre slows down the absorption of carbohydrates, blunting the rate at which blood glucose levels rise and can reduce levels of cholesterol.

INSOLUBLE FIBRE is found in cereals, wholegrains, the skins of vegetables (e.g. potatoes), nuts and seeds. This type of fibre adds bulk to the stool and prevents constipation. 💩

How much do you need?

Your carbohydrate requirement will depend on your activity level as it is the key fuel source for exercise. For example, someone with a sedentary job that involves spending most of the day at a desk will require less carbohydrate than a PE teacher who is running around all day. One size does not fit all, so you need to tune into your body and establish its needs. What I will say is, try opting for a portion of the most nutritionally dense carbohydrates (those that are lower in free sugars – see box on right – and higher in fibre) with your main meals. Examples might include: wholegrains such as brown rice, quinoa and oats; starchy vegetables such as sweet potato and butternut squash; legumes such as beans and lentils; and fruit and vegetables.

What does a serving look like?

- 3–4 heaped tablespoons cooked legumes (beans, peas, lentils)

- 3–4 tablespoons or a clenched fist of cooked wholegrain (oats, rice, quinoa)

- 1–2 slices of bread (opt for wholegrain, brown or seeded for extra fibre)

- 1 baked white or sweet potato, or 3 tablespoons of mash

Of course, fruits and vegetables are carbohydrates too, but they should be included in addition to a portion of those listed above (see pages 136–137 for more information about fruit and veg).

WHAT ARE FREE SUGARS?

I think 'free sugars' is such a misnomer. There's nothing free about them, but that's the term now being used, so I have to stick with it.

The government advises that less than 5% (about 30g) of our daily calories should come from free sugars, which are those added to food and drinks by manufacturers, cooks or consumers, but also includes 'natural' sugars found in honey, syrups and juices. This last category does not include sugars found in fruit and vegetables, grains and cereals, or the lactose naturally present in milk and dairy products.

Free sugars are those we generally need to eat less of as they can contribute to excess calories in our diet and tooth decay. When we see 'total sugars' or 'of which sugars' on a food label, the figure includes both free sugars and natural sugars, so it can be quite confusing. Checking the ingredient list is a good way to spot sugars added to products.

ARE NATURAL SUGARS BETTER THAN REFINED SUGARS?

If you come across health products or foods labelled 'refined sugar free' or 'made with natural sugars', don't be fooled. Whichever sugar you consume, whether it is pure organic honey or pure white sugar, will be handled in the same way by your body, so we should still eat them in moderation. The good news, however, is that sugar present in fruit is packaged up in fibre, which slows the rate at which it is absorbed, so you're less likely to have a rapid spike in blood sugar.

BLOOD GLUCOSE LEVELS

When we talk about blood sugars, we are referring to glucose in the blood. After eating carbohydrates, the body breaks them down into units of glucose. When blood glucose levels rise, cells in the pancreas (a gland that sits underneath the stomach) release a hormone known as insulin. Essentially, insulin acts as a gatekeeper, allowing cells to take up glucose from the blood and use it for energy. As the cells absorb glucose from the blood, levels start to fall. In somebody without diabetes, hormonal mechanisms ensure that these levels never drop too low and stay within a normal range.

Diabetes

In someone suffering from type 1 diabetes, the body does not make any insulin, while someone with type 2 diabetes does not make enough insulin, or the body cannot use the insulin it has as well as it should. In both cases, this causes blood glucose levels to rise because the glucose is unable to access the cells that require it. This results in feelings of tiredness because the cells are energy-starved. The excess glucose in the bloodstream is filtered by the kidneys into the urine, which draws a lot of water with it. This leads to symptoms of excessive urination and thirst. Urine that contains a lot of glucose makes it very easy for bacteria to thrive, so other common symptoms of diabetes are thrush or genital itching. Another effect of high glucose levels in the blood is that wounds take longer to heal and are more prone to infection.

When referring to diabetes, we generally mean type 1 and type 2, but there are other less common forms, such as gestational diabetes, which occurs during pregnancy, and maturity onset diabetes of the young (MODY), which is a rare genetic form.

Type 1 diabetes accounts for 10% of cases in the UK. It is an autoimmune condition, where the immune system mistakes healthy body tissue as a threat and attacks it. In this case, it attacks the cells in the pancreas. The damaged pancreatic cells can't produce insulin, so type 1 diabetics must have daily insulin injections and be aware of how much carbohydrate they consume to match this. While more common in children and teenagers, type 1 diabetes can occur at any age. It cannot be prevented by lifestyle measures.

Type 2 diabetes occurs in 90% of the 3.8 million people that have been diagnosed with diabetes in England. It is also estimated that a further 1.1 million people have diabetes and don't even know it. Type 2 diabetes tends to occur after the age of forty, although more and more people each year are being diagnosed at a younger age. The likelihood of developing this form of diabetes increases with age, obesity, physical inactivity and a positive family history, and is also more common among those of South Asian and Afro-Caribbean ethnicity.

The disease can lead to serious complications, including foot amputation and kidney disease, and is associated with an increased risk of stroke and heart attack. Developing type 2 diabetes is not an inevitable part of ageing, and we have the opportunity to help prevent it from occurring through lifestyle measures.

Tips to reduce the likelihood of developing type 2 diabetes

- Try to move every day – take the stairs, walk the dog or sign up to a fitness class.

- Choose nutrient-dense carbohydrates, e.g. fruits, vegetables, wholegrains and legumes.

- Increase fibre in your diet.

- Include healthy monounsaturated and polyunsaturated fats in your diet.

- Reduce your alcohol consumption.

- Reduce your intake of free sugars and sugar-sweetened beverages.

- If you're concerned that you're at risk, talk to your GP and get your blood glucose levels checked.

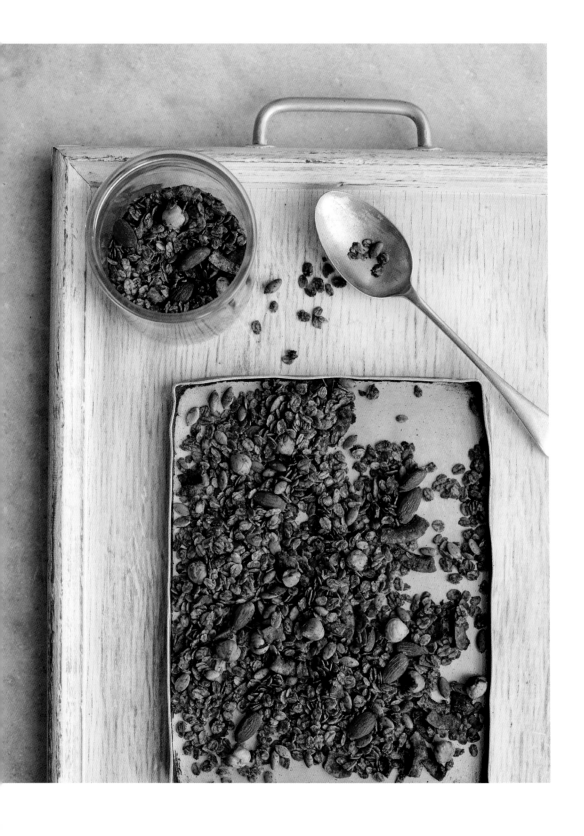

CHOCOLATE ORANGE GRANOLA

SERVES 6–8

Delicious and incredibly easy to make, this granola is also relatively low in sugar compared to the products available in supermarkets. I like to serve my granola with kefir, which is a fermented milk drink that contains beneficial probiotic bacteria, but I also love it spooned on top of yogurt or simply with some cold milk.

200g oats

60g mixed almonds
and hazelnuts

30g pumpkin seeds

30g coconut chips

Zest of 1 orange

1 tsp salt

60ml maple syrup

1 tsp vanilla extract

80ml coconut oil, melted

1 tbsp cocoa powder

Preheat the oven to 160°C/325°F/gas mark 3 and line a baking tray with baking parchment.

Place the oats in a bowl and add the nuts, pumpkin seeds, coconut chips, orange zest and salt.

Combine the remaining ingredients in a separate bowl, then pour into the oat mixture and stir well.

Spread out the mixture on your prepared baking sheet and bake for 40 minutes, stirring gently every 10–15 minutes, or until the oats are golden brown.

Let the granola cool completely on the baking tray before storing it in an airtight container for up to 2 weeks.

MORNING MOCHA SMOOTHIE

SERVES 1

Coffee and breakfast all in one. This is perfect for those who don't like a big breakfast but need their coffee hit. I like to have this if I'm working out early in the morning as it gives me a little boost without leaving me feeling sluggish.

1 frozen banana (see tip), chopped into chunks

40ml cooled espresso or strong coffee (omit for a child-friendly version)

250ml milk

1 tbsp cocoa powder

3 pitted dates

½ tsp vanilla extract

Handful of ice

Place all the ingredients in a blender and blitz until smooth.

TIP: *To freeze a banana, strip off the peel and chop the flesh into small pieces. Place in a sandwich bag or plastic box and pop in the freezer.*

FROZEN STRAWBERRY + PEACH SMOOTHIE

SERVES 1

This smoothie reminds me of Petits Filous yogurt – fruity, creamy and delicious. It's good for grown-ups and kids alike.

80g frozen strawberries

1 peach, chopped

200ml milk

75g natural Greek yogurt

2 tsp maple syrup or honey

Handful of ice cubes

Place all the ingredients in a blender and blitz until smooth.

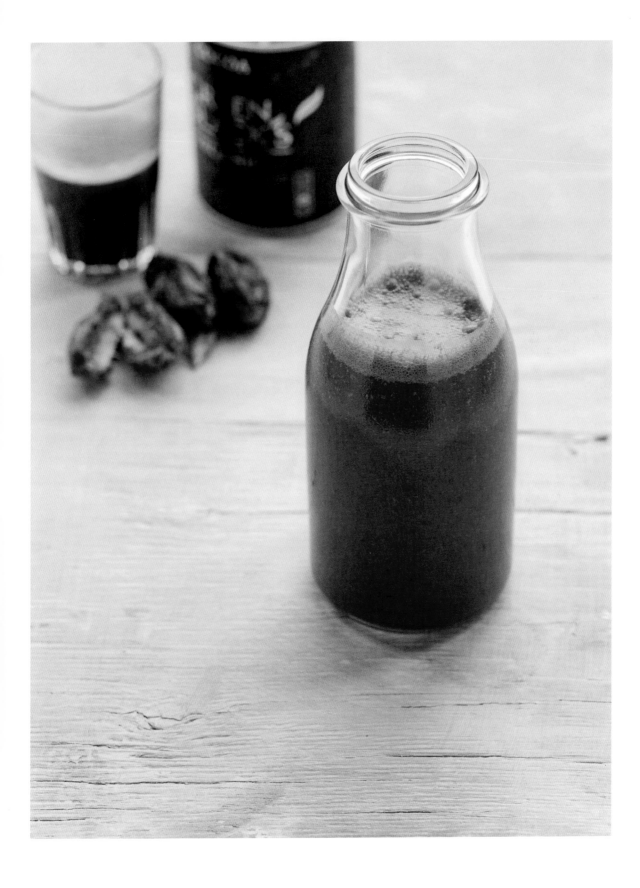

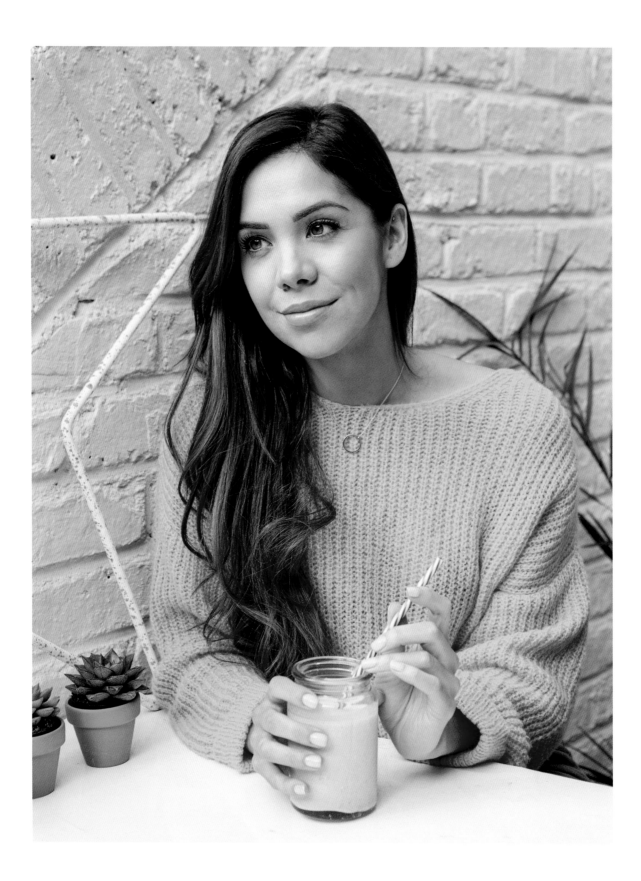

BANANA + FLAX POWER-UP SMOOTHIE

SERVES 1

Thick, creamy and super-satisfying, this smoothie is one of my favourite breakfasts on the go, but also makes a great snack after working out, as it keeps me going until my next meal. It's also great for children or teens before school as it's high in calcium and essential fatty acids – plus it tastes just like a banana milkshake.

1 frozen banana (see tip, page 48)

1 tbsp almond butter or peanut butter

1 tbsp ground flaxseed

200ml milk

¼ tsp vanilla extract

Drizzle of honey or maple syrup

Ground cinnamon

Place all the ingredients, apart from the cinnamon, in a blender and blitz until smooth. Sprinkle with the cinnamon and serve.

DIY YOGURT POTS

I love taking a pot of yogurt and transforming it into something magnificent with crunchy nuts, stewed or caramelised fruit, toasted nuts and honey. Although designed as a convenient breakfast, they're also good enough for dessert. Just saying . . .

TOASTED OAT, QUINOA + STEWED APPLE YOGURT POT

SERVES 1

1 apple, cored and cut into small chunks

1 tbsp coconut sugar or brown sugar

2 tbsp water

1 tsp ground cinnamon

30g oats

1 tbsp uncooked quinoa

200g natural yogurt

Maple syrup, to serve

Put the apple, sugar and water in a small saucepan and bring to a boil. Lower the heat and simmer for 8–10 minutes, until the apples are soft but a few whole chunks still remain. Stir in the cinnamon.

Toast the oats in a dry frying pan over a medium heat for 3–4 minutes, stirring with a wooden spoon. Once they begin to turn golden, add the quinoa and cook for a further minute. Remove from the heat and transfer to a bowl or plate to cool.

Add the yogurt to a jar and top with the apples, cooled oat mixture and a drizzle of maple syrup.

CARAMELISED BANANA + TOASTED NUT YOGURT POT

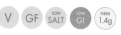

SERVES 1

Handful (about 30g) of nuts

1 banana

½ tbsp coconut oil

1 tbsp honey or maple syrup, plus extra to drizzle

200g natural yogurt

Preheat the oven to 180°C/350°F/gas mark 4.

Line a baking tray with baking parchment and spread the nuts on it in a single layer. Place in the oven for 5–10 minutes, until the nuts darken a couple of shades in colour and begin to give off a lovely nutty aroma. Transfer to a bowl to cool.

Cut the bananas into round slices about 1cm thick. Heat the oil in a frying pan, then stir in the honey. Add the banana and fry over a medium heat for 2–3 minutes, or until the underside starts to brown. Flip the slices over and fry on the other side for another 2–3 minutes.

Place the yogurt in a jar and top with the caramelised banana, the nuts and a drizzle of extra honey.

BLUEBERRY RIPPLE + OAT CRUMBLE YOGURT POT

SERVES 1

1 tsp coconut oil

1 tsp honey or maple syrup

30g jumbo oats

1 tsp desiccated coconut

Pinch of ground cinnamon

200g natural yogurt

2 tbsp Blueberry Chia Jam (see page 241)

Put the coconut oil and honey in a small bowl and melt together in the microwave for 20–30 seconds on full power.

Place the oats, desiccated coconut and cinnamon in a separate bowl. Pour in the hot oil and honey, then stir with a wooden spoon.

Place a non-stick pan over a medium–high heat and toast the oat mixture for 5 minutes, until golden and crunchy. Set aside to cool for 30 minutes.

Spoon half the yogurt into a pot and add a tablespoon of the jam. Add the rest of the yogurt and another spoonful of jam. Swirl a spoon through the mixture to achieve a ripple effect. Sprinkle the oat crumble on top.

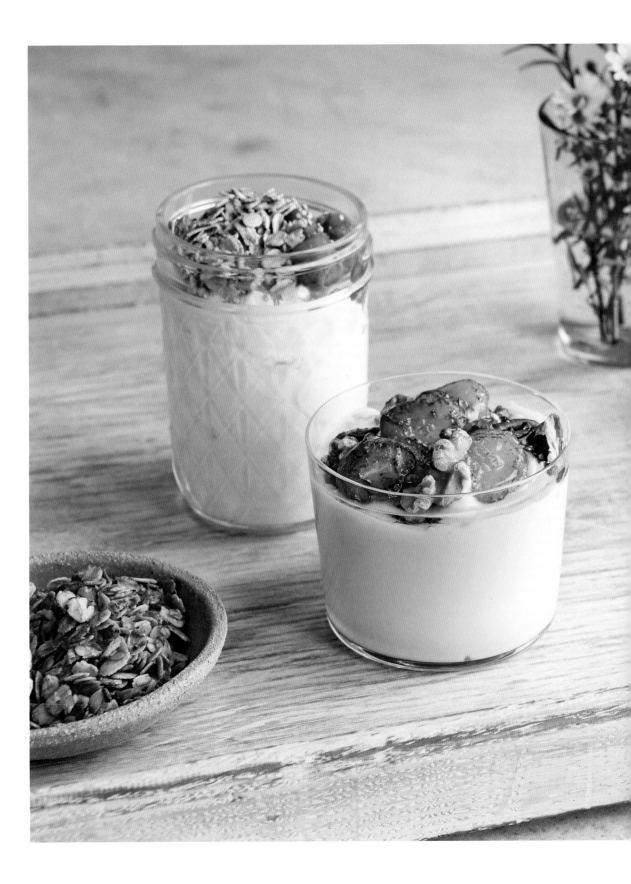

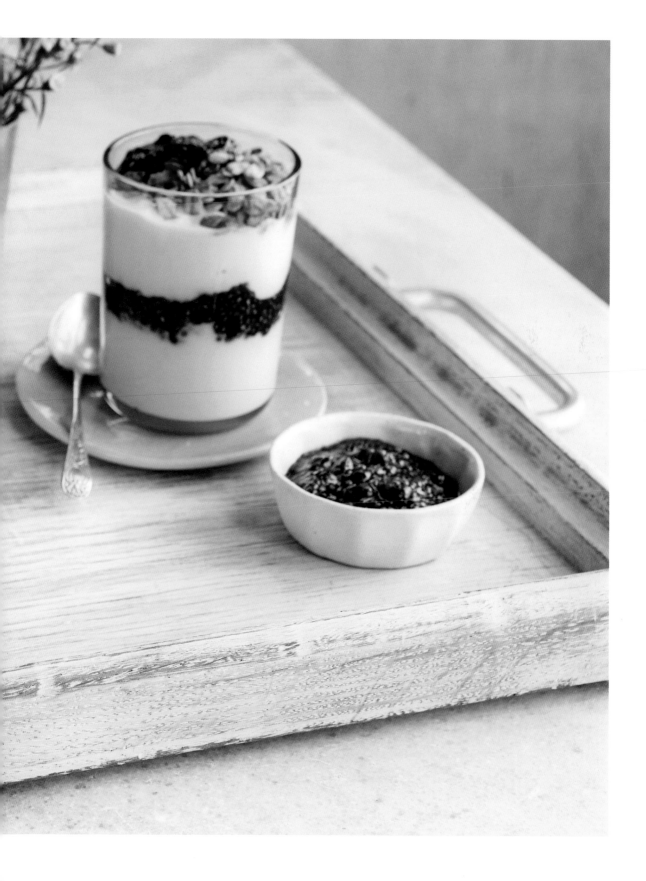

SCRAMBLED EGG, RED PEPPER + CREAM CHEESE PITTA POCKET

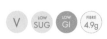

SERVES 1

Here's the perfect fork-free breakfast when you've got a busy day ahead of you and need some rocket fuel!

2 free-range eggs

Dash of milk or water

½ tbsp olive oil

⅓ red bell pepper,
   deseeded and chopped

Handful of spinach

30g cream cheese

Pinch of chilli flakes

1 wholemeal pitta bread

Salt and black pepper

Put the eggs and milk into a small bowl and beat together.

Heat the oil in a medium non-stick frying pan for about 1 minute, then add the red pepper and spinach and cook over a medium–high heat for 1–2 minutes.

Add the egg mixture, cream cheese, chilli flakes and seasoning to the pan. Cook, stirring constantly, for about 1 minute, or until the egg looks just about cooked. Remove from the heat as the egg will continue to cook in the hot pan.

Cut the pitta in half and toast it. Spoon the spinach mixture into the pitta pockets and eat immediately.

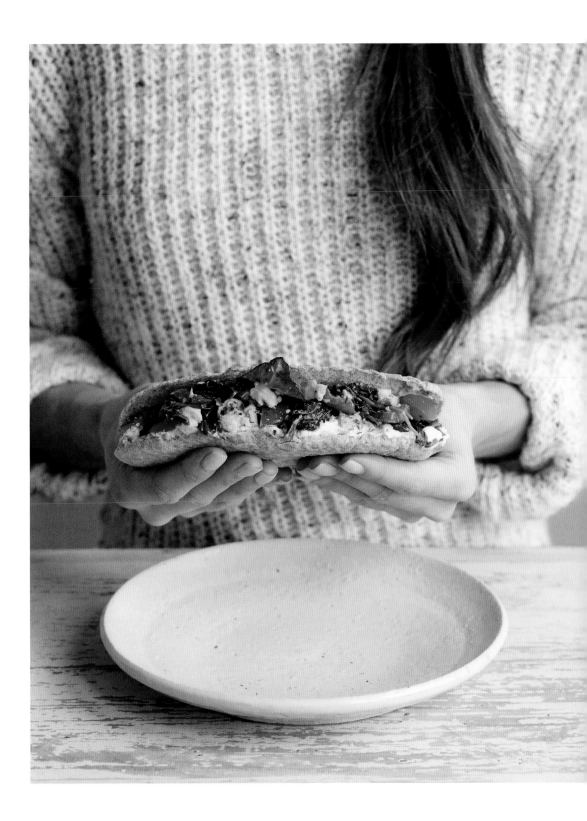

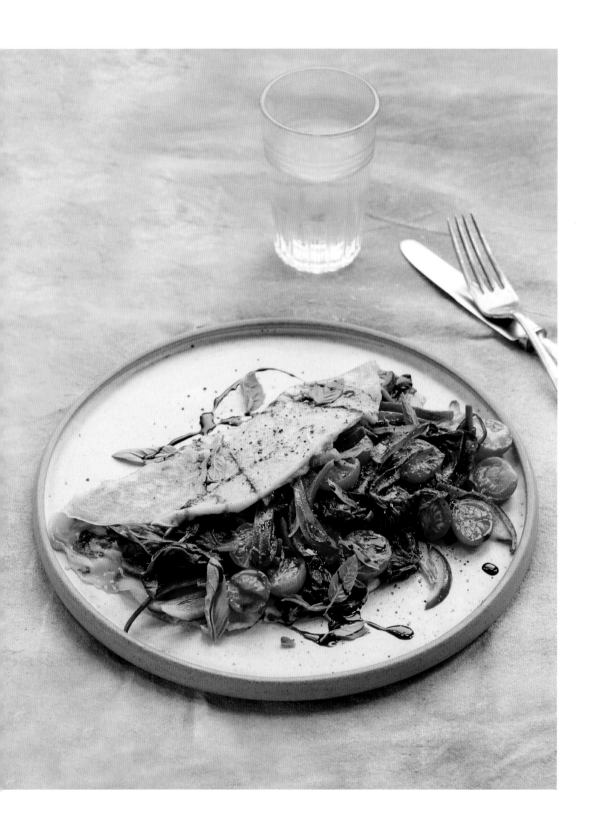

DRESSED-UP TOMATO + CHEESE OMELETTE

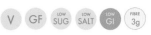

SERVES 1

When I was growing up, I thought an omelette was the most boring thing in the world. There was only so much a girl could take of ham and cheese or tomato and cheese omelettes, so I kind of went off them for a couple of years. As a student, I got back into making them because they're cheap, quick and nutritious. Since then, I've experimented with lots of flavours, fillings and toppings, and now the humble omelette is one of my favourite breakfasts.

3 free-range eggs

Dash of milk or water

1 tbsp freshly chopped basil, or 1 tsp dried basil

1 tbsp butter or olive oil

½ red onion, sliced

5 cherry tomatoes, halved

Handful of spinach

1 tbsp freshly grated Parmesan cheese

Salt and black pepper

Fresh basil leaves, to serve

Balsamic glaze, to drizzle (optional)

Put the eggs, milk and herbs in a bowl and whisk together.

Heat a non-stick frying pan over medium–high heat. Add the butter and swirl to coat the bottom of the pan.

Fry the onion for 3–5 minutes, until soft. Add the tomatoes and spinach. Cook for another minute before adding the egg mixture. Season with salt and pepper.

When the omelette is cooked on the underside, sprinkle the Parmesan on top and fold it in half before sliding it out of the pan (or see tip below).

Tear the basil leaves and sprinkle them on top, add a drizzle of balsamic glaze (if using) and serve immediately.

TIP: *If you don't feel confident folding or rolling the omelette, pop it under a preheated grill for 1–2 minutes instead to cook the top.*

CARROT + APPLE
BREAKFAST MUFFINS

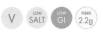

MAKES 12

One way to make sure you're hitting your five-a-day is sneaking fruit and vegetables into a muffin, right? Perfect for breakfast, snacking or even dessert, these veggie-packed muffins are good at any time of day.

1 cooking apple, peeled, cored and diced

3 tbsp water

150g carrot, peeled and coarsely grated

250g white spelt flour

50g wholegrain spelt flour

1 tsp baking powder

1 tsp bicarbonate of soda

1 tsp mixed spice

pinch of salt

2 free-range eggs, beaten

140ml natural yogurt

200ml maple syrup

1 eating apple, peeled, cored and diced

Preheat the oven to 200°C/400°F/gas mark 6. Grease and line a 12-hole muffin tray.

Place the cooking apple in a small saucepan with the water. Bring to the boil, then simmer for 5 minutes, until the apple is completely soft. Mash with a fork, then mix in the carrot and set aside to cool.

Put both spelt flours in a large bowl, add the baking powder, bicarbonate of soda, the mixed spice and salt and stir together.

Add the eggs, yogurt, maple syrup, mashed apple mixture and the diced apple. Stir well.

Divide the mixture between the muffin cases and bake for 15–20 minutes, or until a skewer comes out mostly clean. (These muffins are moist, so there may be a few crumbs clinging to the skewer even when fully baked.)

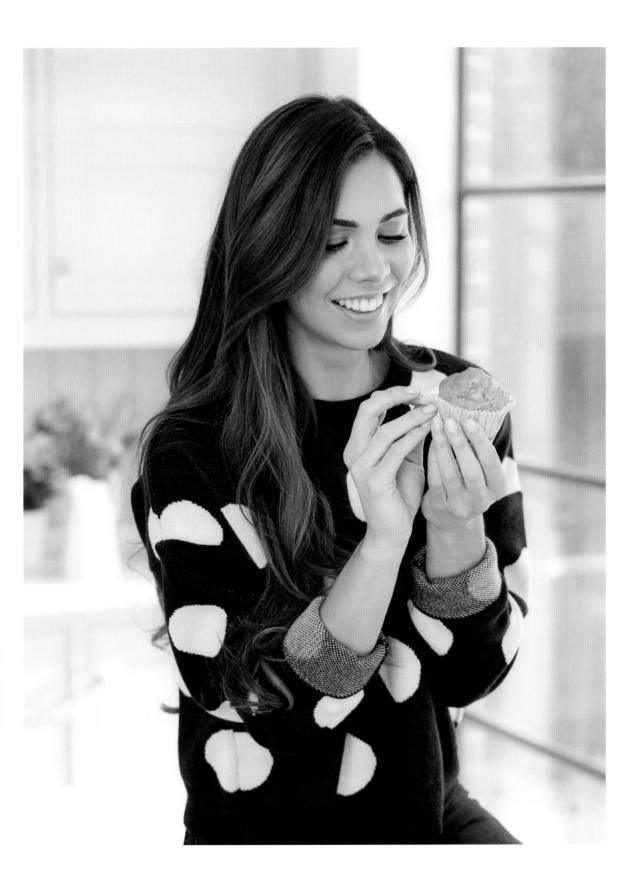

CRANBERRY + PECAN
GRANOLA BARS

MAKES 18–20

*These are the ultimate grab-and-go bars with a flask of coffee –
perfect for those mornings when you've snoozed one too many times.
If cranberries aren't your thing, try other dried fruit, such as raisins
or chopped apricots. Similarly, you can use any nuts you wish.*

280g oats (not jumbo oats)
160g medjool dates, pitted
100g soft unsalted butter
100g dried cranberries
100g pecan nuts, roughly
    chopped
Finely grated zest of
    ½ orange
¼ tsp salt

Preheat the oven to 160°C/325°F/gas mark 3. Grease and line
a shallow baking tin (18 x 24cm) with baking parchment.

Spread the oats out in a baking tray and toast in the oven for
10 minutes, until lightly browned.

Meanwhile, place the dates and butter in a blender or food processor
and blitz until completely smooth.

Put the toasted oats in a large bowl and add the date mixture,
cranberries, pecans, orange zest and salt. Mix well, then spread the
mixture into the prepared tin, using the back of a spoon to compact
it firmly and ensure it is flat.

Bake for 35–40 minutes, until golden and slightly crispy. Set aside to
cool, then cut into bars. Store in an airtight container for up to a week.

LUNCH ON THE RUN

It is no secret that I am the self-proclaimed queen of the lunchbox. After the publication of my first book, I asked readers what they wanted to see more of and the resounding response was for lunchbox recipes. I actually thought about doing a cookbook purely on portable lunches, but thought that I might as well go the whole nine yards and do breakfast, lunch and dinner – and snacks.

In this chapter you will find inspiration for open sandwiches, your own DIY salad jars, warming soups to serve with chunky slices of bread, plus falafels and burgers of every kind to batch-cook at the weekend and enjoy throughout the week. It's time to reclaim your lunch break and have something to look forward to – something that will brighten even the most stressful of days. My ideas for fresh and sustaining meals will nourish you from the inside out.

REINVENTING THE SALAD

I begrudge paying £5 or £6 for shop-bought salads because they tend to be limp with skimpy amounts of vegetables. Making a salad from scratch, though, gives you the power to make a nutrient-packed, full-of-flavour, low-cost lunch that you're actually excited to have.

The word 'salad' is often associated with negative connotations, such as 'rabbit food', 'unsatisfying' and 'boring'. If these are some of the words that spring to mind when you think about salad, I want to reframe your thoughts. And part of that is to stop thinking of 'salad' as interchangeable with 'lettuce'. Let me make it clear: the base of every salad does not need to be lettuce or leafy greens, and when it is, there are far more options than iceberg. Think about chicory, radicchio, watercress, rocket and lambs' lettuce. Each adds its own distinctive flavour and texture to the salad.

Now that I've finished ranting, let me show you how to fall in love with salads again.

PICK + MIX SALAD JARS

THE QUANTITIES ALL PROVIDE ONE SERVING.

If you have a copy of my first book, you'll probably remember the pick 'n' mix approach in my Shakes and Smoothies section. It became a huge favourite with everyone, perhaps because we all love variety and excitement in our lives.

I like to layer my salads in big clip-top jars, but you can serve yours simply on a plate or in a lunchbox. Layered salad jars just look visually appealing, and the clever layering will help to keep your salad fresh and crunchy until lunchtime.

Below is a guide to how it works. The vegetables and ingredients I list are just examples, generally those that are easy to find in most supermarkets. However, do feel free to add different things that you particularly enjoy.

LAYER 1 – DRESSING: This is the liquid layer and needs to be at the bottom of the jar. (See opposite page for some simple salad dressings.)

LAYER 2 – CRUNCHY VEGETABLES: I like to add these on top of the dressing so that they can soften a little. Choose from bell peppers, celery, onion, broccoli, asparagus, edamame beans, radishes, grated carrot and green beans.

LAYER 3 – COMPLEX CARBOHYDRATES: These are your starchy vegetables, wholegrains and legumes, which provide you with energy. Choose from brown or wild rice, quinoa, freekah, millet, farro, barley, buckwheat, noodles, lentils, chickpeas, beans, sweet potato, white potato and butternut squash.

LAYER 4 – PROTEIN: This will keep you feeling fuller for longer so that you can keep going until dinnertime. Choose from feta or goat's cheese, roast chicken or turkey, salmon or mackerel, tinned tuna, sardines or anchovies, prawns, or hard-boiled eggs. If you're vegan, add tofu or another portion of beans, peas or lentils to get your full protein hit.

LAYER 5 – SOFT VEGETABLES: These are veg that get soggy quickly, so placing them near the top means they will be protected from the moisture in the other layers and retain their bite. Choose from beetroot, roasted aubergine, roasted peppers, grilled courgettes, sweetcorn, avocado, spring onions, marinated artichokes and sundried tomatoes.

LAYER 6 – ACCESSORIES: This is the fun layer, where you can boost the taste and texture of the entire jar. Choose from pomegranate seeds, olives, hummus, salsa, guacamole, fermented foods such as sauerkraut and kimchi, mango, nuts and seeds, lentil sprouts and fresh herbs.

LAYER 7 – LEAFY GREENS: The delicate greens go at the very top to prevent them from becoming soggy. Choose from kale, rocket, spinach, watercress, chicory, pak choi, romaine or baby gem lettuce.

PICK + MIX SALAD DRESSINGS

BALSAMIC DRESSING	HONEY MUSTARD DRESSING	SOY DRESSING	TAHINI DRESSING
3 tbsp extra-virgin olive oil	3 tbsp extra-virgin olive oil	4 tbsp olive oil	3 tbsp tahini
1 tbsp balsamic vinegar	2 tbsp white wine vinegar	1 tbsp soy sauce	2 tbsp lemon juice
1 garlic clove, peeled and grated	1 tsp Dijon mustard	Juice of ½ lemon	1 tbsp apple cider vinegar
Pinch of dried Italian herbs (optional)	2 tsp honey	1 garlic clove, peeled and grated	2 garlic cloves, peeled and grated
Salt and black pepper	Salt and black pepper	1 tsp sugar	1 tbsp maple syrup
		Salt and black pepper	50–60ml water
			Salt and black pepper

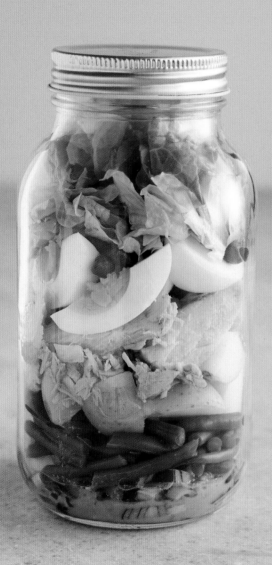

THE
FRENCH
ONE

2 tbsp Honey Mustard
  Dressing (optional,
  see page 65)

1 tbsp chopped red onion

Handful of green beans,
  blanched in boiling
  water for 2 minutes

3 baby potatoes, boiled
  and quartered

1 x 80g tin of tuna
  or salmon

1 hard-boiled free-range
  egg, halved

1 tbsp capers

Romaine lettuce

 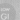

GF   LOW SUG   LOW GI   FIBRE 6.0g

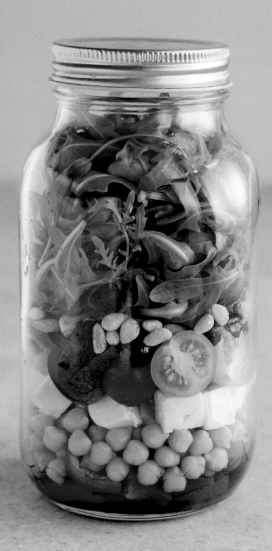

THE ITALIAN ONE

2 tbsp Balsamic Dressing (optional, see page 65)

½ red pepper, deseeded and diced

3 tbsp chickpeas, rinsed and drained

50g feta cheese, cut into cubes

4 cherry tomatoes, halved

4–5 pitted black olives, sliced

1 tbsp pine nuts

Handful of rocket leaves

V · GF · LOW SUG · LOW GI · FIBRE 6.2g

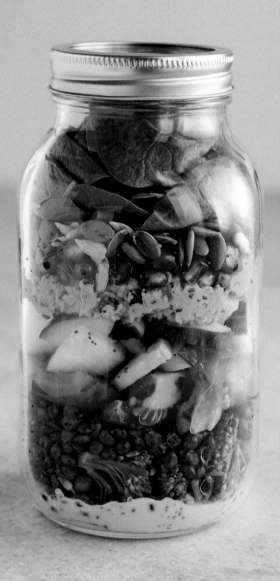

THE MIDDLE EASTERN ONE

2 tbsp Tahini Dressing (optional, see page 65)

Handful of broccoli, chopped into small pieces

3 tbsp cooked lentils

1 salad tomato, chopped

¼ cucumber, chopped

Dollop of Baked Aubergine Hummus (optional, see page 130)

1 tbsp pomegranate seeds

1 tbsp mixed seeds, e.g. sunflower, sesame, etc.

Handful of fresh baby spinach

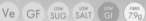 Ve · GF · LOW SUG · LOW SALT · LOW GI · FIBRE 7.9g

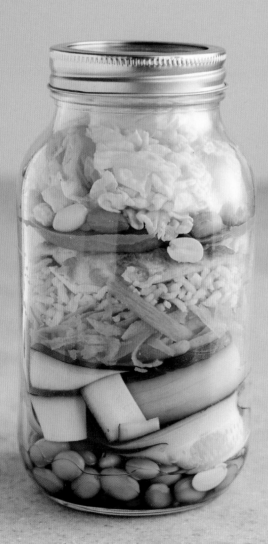

THE
ASIAN
ONE

2 tbsp Soy Dressing
(optional, see page 65)

2 tbsp edamame beans

1 small courgette, shaved
into ribbons

½ carrot, peeled
and grated

3 tbsp brown rice

100g chicken breast,
torn into pieces

¼ avocado, sliced

1 tbsp peanuts

Handful of pak choi,
chopped

LOW SUG LOW SALT LOW GI FIBRE 7.1g

REINVENTING THE SANDWICH

We have let the sandwich down. I'm sorry to say that it has become the least appetising thing on the lunch menu. I really do not want flabby white bread with a slice of rubbery cheese in the middle; and offering me a packet of crisps and a chocolate bar as part of the deal does not make it taste any better (well, maybe a little). It's time to save your pennies and fall back in love with homemade sandwiches.

As the top slice of the sandwich is generally missing out on all the action, I like to have open sandwiches as you can add more toppings.

- **CHOOSE FRESH, NUTTY, WHOLEGRAIN OR SOURDOUGH BREAD** rather than a standard sliced loaf.

- **LOAD IT UP WITH TASTY FATS** such as hummus, avocado, nut butter and cheese.

- **PILE IT HIGH WITH LEAFY GREENS** and colourful vegetables that make you want to Instagram the hell out of it!

- **PACK IT WITH PROTEIN** to keep you full and satisfied so you don't need that packet of crisps to fill the gap.

Here are some of my favourite combinations.

OPEN SANDWICH WITH TURKEY, APPLE + BRIE

SERVES 1

2 slices of sourdough bread

1–2 tsp Dijon mustard

Handful of rocket leaves

100g roast turkey breast

4 slices of Brie cheese

½ green apple, cored
and thinly sliced

Place the bread on a board and spread each slice with mustard.

Top with the rocket leaves, followed by the turkey, Brie and apple slices.

OPEN SANDWICH WITH BEETROOT, MINT + TAHINI DIP + FLAKED SALMON

SERVES 1

2 slices of rye bread,
shop-bought or
homemade (see
page 211)

2 tbsp Beetroot, Mint
and Tahini Dip (see
page 130)

1 cooked salmon fillet

Mint leaves, to serve
(optional)

Place the bread on a board and spread each slice with the dip.

Flake the salmon fillet and scatter over the top. Tear the mint leaves and sprinkle them over the fish.

OPEN SANDWICH WITH BAKED AUBERGINE HUMMUS + ROASTED PEPPERS

SERVES 1

2 slices of sourdough bread

2 tbsp Baked Aubergine Hummus (see page 130)

100g roasted red peppers, shop-bought or homemade, drained

1 tbsp toasted seeds, e.g. sunflower, sesame, etc.

Place the bread on a board and spread each slice with the hummus.

Roughly chop the peppers and place them on top. Sprinkle with the seeds.

OPEN SANDWICH WITH PEANUT BUTTER, STRAWBERRIES + HONEY

SERVES 1

2 slices of rye bread, shop-bought or homemade (see page 211)

2 tbsp peanut butter

5–6 strawberries, sliced

Honey, to drizzle

Toast the bread, then spread the peanut butter on each slice.

Top with the strawberries and drizzle with honey.

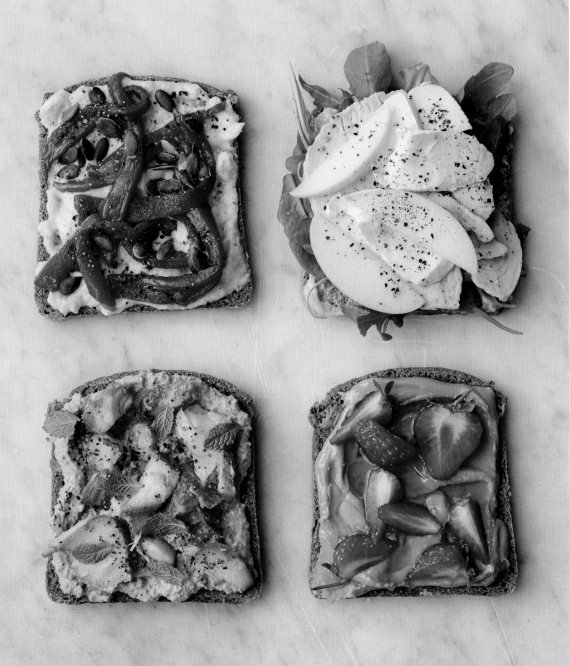

SOUPS

Soup has to be my ultimate comfort food, especially when served with some freshly baked bread for dunking! I love how versatile it is and how easily you can pack a whole load of goodness into a single bowl. I've included a few of my favourite recipes here but feel free to experiment with some of your favourite vegetables, grains, herbs and spices to create your own concoctions.

LENTIL SOUP

SERVES 4–6

This soup is hearty, filling and comforting, made with ingredients that you most likely already have in your store cupboard.

3 tbsp olive oil, plus extra to drizzle

2 onions, finely chopped

4 garlic cloves, crushed

2 tsp ground cumin

½ tsp ground turmeric

½ tsp ground coriander

½ teaspoon salt

1 litre vegetable stock

200g uncooked green or Puy lentils, washed and drained

200ml water

Salt and black pepper

Small handful of chopped parsley, to serve

Put the olive oil in a saucepan and place over a medium heat. When hot, add the onions, garlic, spices and ½ teaspoon salt and sauté for 10 minutes, until the onions are translucent and soft.

Add the stock, lentils and water, bring to the boil, then cover and simmer for 40–45 minutes, until the lentils are cooked through and the soup is thick. Taste and adjust the seasoning if necessary.

Serve in bowls with the parsley scattered over and an extra drizzle of oil.

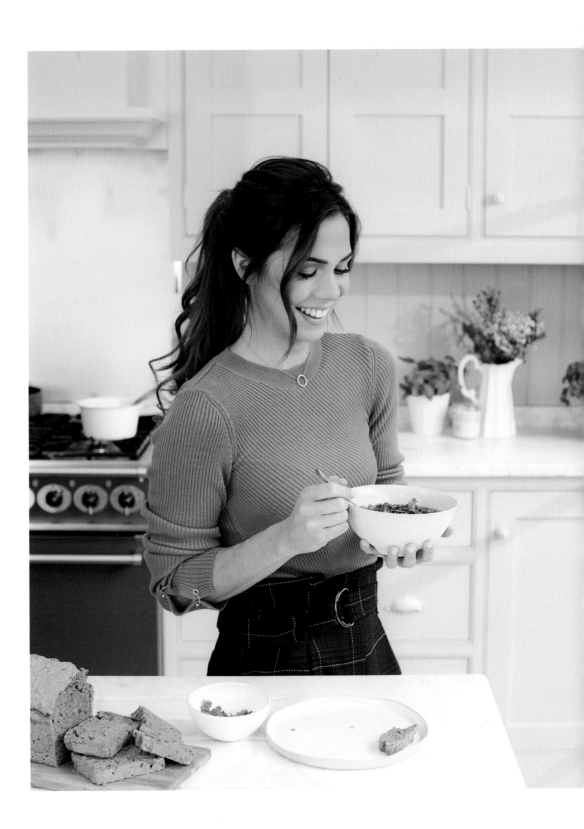

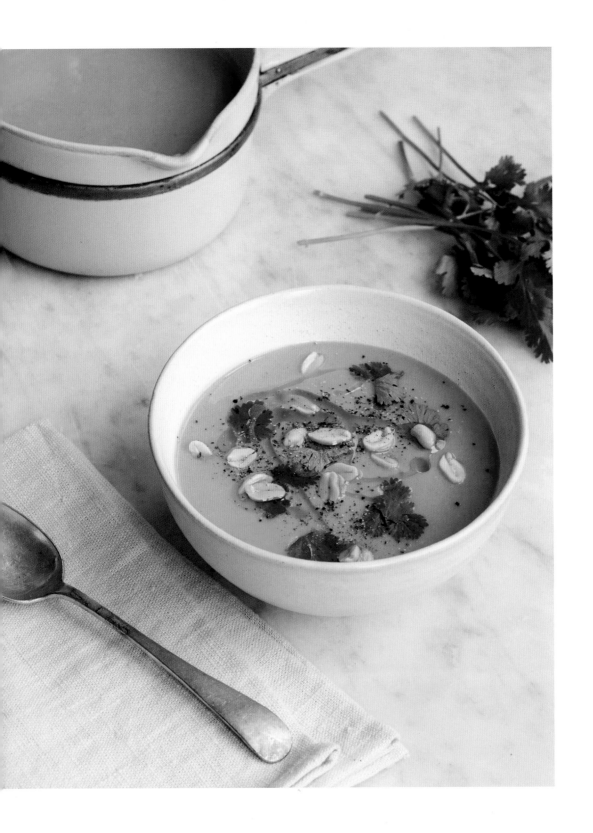

SPICY SWEET POTATO + PEANUT BUTTER SOUP

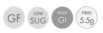

SERVES 4–5

By now you must think that I'm obsessed with peanut butter. Well, you're right – I am! Jokes aside, it really works well in this savoury dish and adds a lovely nutty undertone. This is a super-filling soup with a bit of a kick, so perfect for those chilly days at work when you need a hug in a mug.

1¼ tbsp coconut oil

1 onion, diced

2 garlic cloves, chopped

½ tsp ground cumin

2 tbsp red curry paste

2 tbsp creamy peanut butter or almond butter

1 litre vegetable stock

2 sweet potatoes (about 600g in total), peeled and cubed

½ tsp salt, plus extra salt and pepper to adjust seasoning

Handful of roasted peanuts, chopped (optional)

Chopped coriander (optional)

Place the oil in a large saucepan (the biggest you have) over a medium heat. When hot, fry the onion and garlic for 5 minutes until soft and translucent.

Lower the heat, then stir in the cumin, curry paste and peanut butter. Stirring constantly, slowly pour in the stock, stirring to combine.

Add the sweet potatoes and salt and bring to the boil. Cover and simmer for 20 minutes, until the potato is soft.

Remove from the heat and use a hand blender to blitz until smooth and creamy. If you don't have a hand blender, allow the soup to cool for 20 minutes, then blitz the soup in a food processor or blender in small batches. The finished soup should be thick and creamy, but if it is too thick for your liking, simply add a small amount of water and blend to combine.

Taste and season with salt and black pepper if necessary. Ladle the soup into bowls and serve sprinkled with the peanuts and coriander, if you wish.

SERENA'S VEGETABLE SOUP

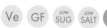

SERVES 4–6

Serena is my best friend's mum, and she's been best friends with my own mum ever since we were little, so I spent a lot of time in her house when growing up. Serena used to make her vegetable soup when we got in from school and would serve it with warm bread rolls filled with slices of Cheddar. This is the soup I dream of when I'm missing home. It's very easy to make and you can use whatever root vegetables you wish. For a change, Serena says you can use tomato pesto instead of tomato purée.

2 tbsp olive oil

1 kg peeled and chopped vegetables, e.g. large onion, celery, carrot, parsnip, potato)

1 litre vegetable stock

1 x 400g tin of chopped tomatoes

1 tbsp tomato purée

1 tsp mixed dried herbs

Salt and black pepper

Heat the oil in a large saucepan and fry the onion for 4–5 minutes, until soft. Add the rest of the vegetables and fry for 5 minutes, stirring to ensure they don't burn. Cover and sweat the vegetables over a low heat for 10 minutes or so.

Add the stock and remaining ingredients. Bring to the boil, then simmer for 30–40 minutes, until the vegetables are soft.

Blend the soup until smooth. Season with salt and pepper.

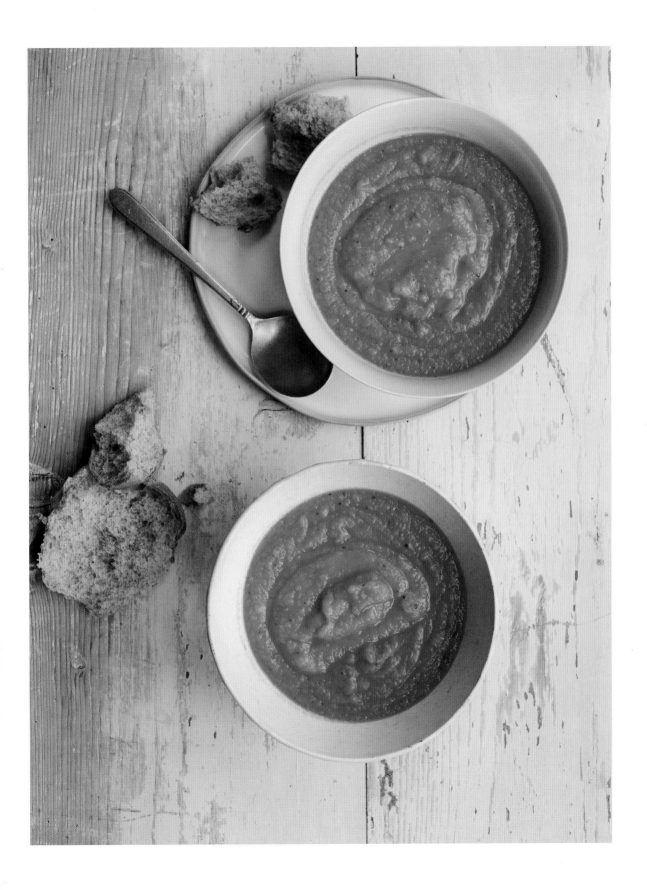

MICRONUTRIENTS

Micronutrients include vitamins and minerals, which are essential nutrients that your body needs in small amounts. Phytonutrients are a third group of nutrients, which are non-essential for life but offer beneficial effects on health.

The amount of vitamins and minerals you need varies depending on age, where you're from and where you live, your gender and, for women, whether you are pregnant, breastfeeding or post-menopausal.

In theory, we should be able to get all our essential nutrients through a well-balanced diet, with one exception – vitamin D!

VITAMIN D

This essential vitamin is made in the skin following exposure to sunshine, and is important for healthy bones and teeth. A deficiency can lead to rickets in children, or the adult version, osteomalacia, where the bones soften and become weak.

Current advice in the UK from Public Health England (PHE) is that children over the age of one and all adults should take a 10 microgram supplement of vitamin D each day throughout autumn and winter. This is because it is difficult to make enough from the amount of sunlight there is in this part of the world, and it's hard to get enough from diet alone. However, during spring and summer, the majority of us will get enough vitamin D.

Certain groups of people may need to take a vitamin D supplement all year round, namely:

- People who spend most of their time indoors, such as those who are housebound or in care homes.

- People who must always have their skin covered.

- Dark-skinned people of African, Afro-Caribbean and South Asian ethnicity may also not get enough vitamin D from sunlight because the pigment (melanin) in dark skin doesn't absorb as much UV radiation.

- Pregnant women and breastfeeding mothers.

- People aged over sixty-five because their skin is less good at making vitamin D.

- Those who do not have diets rich in vitamin D.

The main dietary sources of vitamin D in the UK are animal foods and fortified plant foods. The richest sources include egg yolk, oily fish (e.g. salmon, mackerel, herring, sardines) and meat, but vitamin D is also found in fortified milk, margarine and certain breakfast cereals. For more information on vitamin D and a plant-based diet, see page 164.

CALCIUM

Like vitamin D, calcium has an important role in bone and teeth formation, but it also plays a part in the contraction and relaxation of blood vessels and muscles, and in nerve transmission. Adequate intake of calcium is important at all ages, but even more so for growing kids and teens, when bones are developing, and in later years, particularly in post-menopausal women, when bones start to thin. Absorption of calcium in the gut also depends on vitamin D, so these two nutrients are essential for strong, healthy bones.

Calcium is found in dairy products such as milk, cheese and yogurt, tinned fish (with bones), nuts and seeds, some green vegetables, and fortified foods. If you have a lactose intolerance, or exclude dairy from your diet for any reason, you are more at risk of calcium deficiency. See page 166 to read more about calcium in a plant-based diet.

PHYTONUTRIENTS

In addition to providing vitamins, minerals and fibre, fruit and vegetables are also sources of phytonutrients, aka phytochemicals, the natural protective substances found in plants that often give them their vibrant colours. Although they are not considered essential to the human diet, as they are not absolutely vital for survival, they exhibit antioxidant properties, which may protect against the development and progression of many chronic conditions, including cardiovascular problems and cancer.

Fruits, vegetables, grains, legumes, nuts and tea are all rich sources of phytonutrients, but the amounts vary from plant to plant. It's therefore important not only to increase our consumption of fruit and vegetables in general, but also to increase the variety. There are tens of thousands of phytochemicals, and scientists believe that there are probably many more they haven't yet discovered in the foods we eat.

WHAT ARE ANTIOXIDANTS?

While 'antioxidant' has become a bit of a buzzword, I think many people are hazy about what it actually means, so here goes . . .

Various nutrients and enzymes, such as vitamins C and E, minerals such as zinc and selenium, phytochemicals such as beta-carotene, and enzymes such as glutathione, are all considered antioxidants because of a shared type of property that they exhibit. Basically, they prevent cell damage caused by unstable molecules in the body known as 'free radicals'. Antioxidants combine with and neutralise free radicals, thereby preventing them from causing damage. This is thought to be important because cell damage caused by free radicals has been linked to ageing and degenerative disease. However, this is not true of all antioxidants, and some studies show benefits only in test-tube experiments (as opposed to the human body), but the research is growing and some very exciting findings are being made.

VARIETY IS ESSENTIAL

Both quantity and variety of fruits and vegetables are important to obtain the maximum benefit from the foods we eat. I'm not going to bore you with a list of them, but here are a few that you might already have come across:

CAROTENOIDS are yellow and orange pigments found in carrots, sweetcorn, butternut squash, pumpkins, mangoes and oranges. A few carotenoids are red, such as the lycopene found in tomatoes. All have been extensively researched for their role as antioxidants and their protective role in eye health.

POLYPHENOLS are phytochemicals that contribute to the colour, taste and smell of many foods. There has been a huge interest in polyphenols for their potential role in the prevention of various diseases, particularly cardiovascular disease.

IS DARK CHOCOLATE GOOD FOR YOU?

Ever hear that dark chocolate is good for you? Well, it's all down to a group of polyphenols known as flavonols, which are present in chocolate. Flavonols have attracted a huge amount of interest due to their potential ability to lower blood pressure, a known risk factor for cardiovascular disease. The blood pressure-reducing effects of flavonols are thought to be related to widening of the blood vessels, caused by nitric oxide.

However, before you start reaching for a Snickers bar, note that a review of thirty-five studies found the blood pressure-lowering effect to be very small. So although the research shows some interesting effects, particularly in heart health, I don't think chocolate will be included in dietary guidelines just yet. But that doesn't mean we can't enjoy it as part of a balanced diet. I certainly won't be giving up my daily dose of chocolate.

Finally, do bear in mind that the type of chocolate used in studies is often very different from the chocolate that we pick up at the local shop. So yes, chocolate contains polyphenols but, unlike fruit and vegetables, it also contains fat and sugar. Calorie for calorie, then, fruit and vegetables are for sure a better choice in terms of boosting your phytonutrient intake.

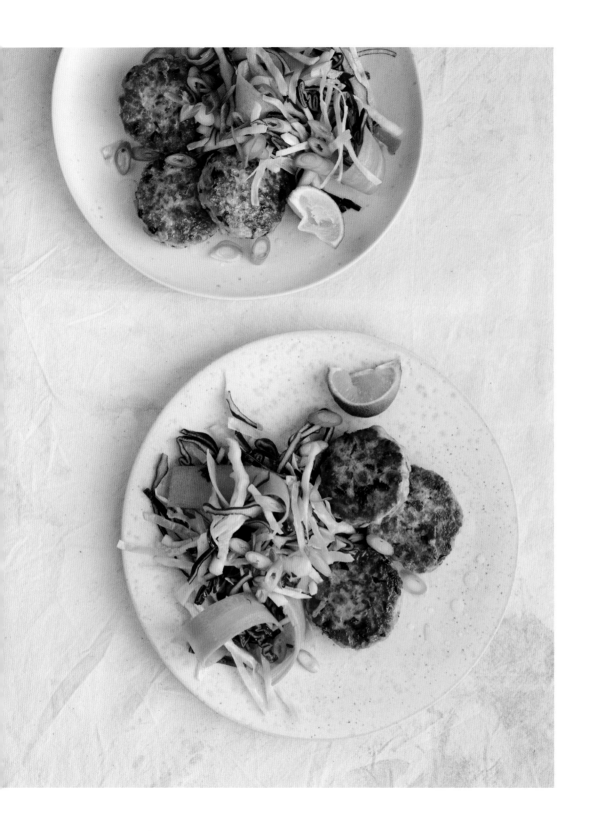

BURGERS AND FALAFELS

Burgers and falafels are the ultimate fork-free foods and make the perfect lunches for when you're on the go, at the office or at home. I love jazzing up the burgers with my favourite toppings, serving them in a crispy bun or with a simple side salad, or with my famous sweet and smoky sweet potato fries (see page 86). Homemade falafel is far more easy than it sounds and tastes absolutely delicious hot or cold, in a salad or in a wrap.

THAI SALMON BURGERS

SERVES 2

It's hard to believe that something so easy to make could be so delicious, but these burgers will persuade even the fussiest of people to eat fish. Salmon is full of omega 3 fatty acids, which are associated with improved mood, brain function and heart health.

2 boneless, skinless salmon fillets

1 tbsp Thai red curry paste

3 tbsp oats

2.5cm piece of fresh root ginger, peeled and grated

Handful of fresh coriander (optional)

1 tbsp coconut oil or olive oil

Lime wedges, to serve

Cut the salmon into chunks and place in a blender or food processor with the curry paste, oats, ginger and coriander (if using). Pulse until roughly minced.

Divide the mixture in half and shape each piece into 6 mini burgers.

Heat the oil in a non-stick frying pan, then fry the burgers for 5 minutes on each side, until golden and cooked through.

Serve with lime wedges and a side of Rainbow Slaw with Asian Vinaigrette (see page 94).

LENTIL + BEETROOT BURGERS

SERVES 4

I used to roll my eyes at people who ordered vegetarian burgers in restaurants. I mean, what's a burger without meat? Well, I was proved wrong, and now I almost always choose a veggie burger rather than a meat burger – unless it's good-quality beef that I just can't pass up on. If you are like I was, and slightly sceptical of the veggie option, I urge you to try this recipe.

2 x 400g tins of green or Puy lentils, drained, or 500g cooked lentils

200g cooked beetroot (see tip below), peeled and coarsely grated

4 spring onions, finely chopped

2 free-range eggs, beaten

3 garlic cloves, crushed

Large handful of flat-leaf parsley leaves, finely chopped

1 tsp ground cumin

1 tsp sweet smoked paprika

100g oats (not jumbo oats)

1½ tsp salt

Black pepper

Olive oil, to fry

TO SERVE

Burger buns or pitta breads

Mayonnaise, mustard, etc.

2 heads of romaine lettuce, leaves separated

½ red onion, thinly sliced

2 beef tomatoes, sliced

Put half the lentils into a blender or food processor and blitz to a purée. Transfer to a large bowl, then add the reserved whole lentils and all the remaining ingredients, except the oil. Stir together.

Preheat the oven to 200°C/400°F/gas mark 6. Line a baking tray with baking parchment.

Divide the lentil mixture into 8 equal pieces and shape them into patties 2cm thick. Add a tablespoon of the oil to a frying pan and set over a low–medium heat. When hot, fry the burgers in batches for 3–4 minutes on each side, until crisp and golden, adding a little more oil if needed. Transfer to the prepared tray and bake for 20 minutes.

Serve the patties in burger buns or pitta bread, with a little mayonnaise or mustard, the lettuce, onion and tomato slices.

TIP: *Most supermarkets sell vacuum-packed cooked beetroot in the fruit and veg section, so I pretty much always buy them in this form because it's so quick and convenient. If you prefer to cook your own, pop the whole (unpeeled) beetroot into a pan of boiling water and let them bubble away for anything from 30 minutes to 1½ hours, depending on size. You will know they're ready when the skin crinkles away from the flesh when you pinch it and they are tender inside when tested with a skewer or pointed knife.*

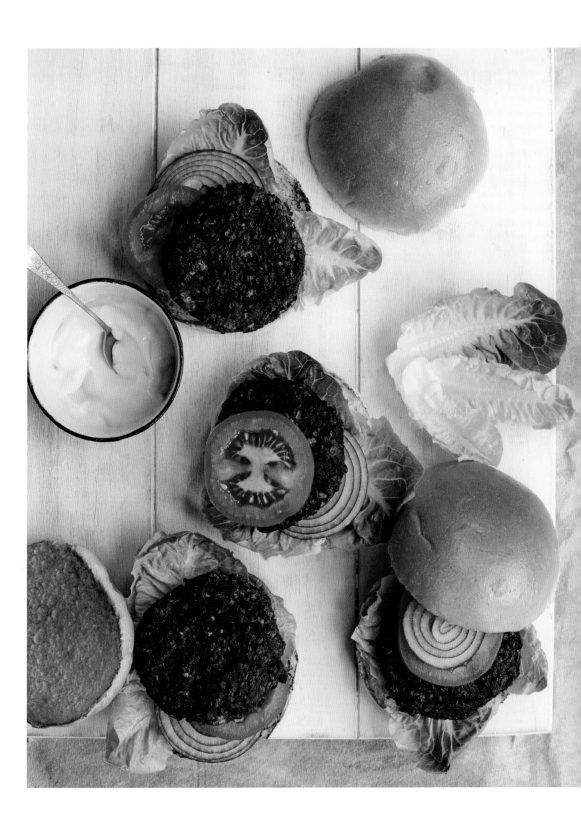

CARROT + CORIANDER CHICKPEA BURGERS WITH TOMATO SALSA + SWEET POTATO FRIES

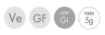

SERVES 4

I love these burgers because they're very similar to falafel, but feel slightly more substantial. I cannot usually stand the taste of coriander, but when it's fresh and blended up in this recipe, it really adds something. I serve the burgers with the easiest tomato salsa in the world, which lifts them from good to awesome.

2–3 tbsp olive oil

1 onion, chopped

2 garlic cloves, grated

1 x 400g tin of chickpeas, drained and rinsed

½ large carrot (about 60g), peeled and grated

Handful of fresh coriander

50g oats

Juice of ½ lime

1 tbsp tahini

1 tsp ground cumin

¼ tsp salt

FOR THE FRIES

2 sweet potatoes, peeled and cut into wedges

1 tbsp olive oil

1 tbsp maple syrup

1 tsp smoked paprika

1 tsp ground cinnamon

Pinch of salt

FOR THE SALSA

2 large tomatoes, finely chopped

½ red onion, diced

1 garlic clove, grated

1 tbsp extra-virgin olive oil

Salt and black pepper

Preheat the oven to 190°C/375°F/gas mark 5. Line 2 baking trays with baking parchment.

First make the fries. Place the sweet potato chunks in a bowl and add all the remaining ingredients for them. Toss well, then place in one of the prepared trays and bake for 35–40 minutes.

Meanwhile, make the burgers. Heat a tablespoon of the oil in a frying pan, then fry the onion and garlic until soft and translucent.

Place the chickpeas in a blender or food processor and add the fried onion and garlic together with all the remaining burger ingredients. Blend for about 1 minute, until combined, but not completely smooth.

Divide the mixture into 4 equal pieces and shape them into patties 2cm thick. Transfer to the prepared tray and bake for 20 minutes. Remove from the oven.

Heat the remaining olive oil in a frying pan and cook the burgers for 2–3 minutes on each side, until golden. This firms them up, so they're less likely to crumble.

Meanwhile, make the salsa. Simply combine the ingredients in a bowl and season to taste with salt and pepper.

Serve the burgers with the salsa and sweet potato fries.

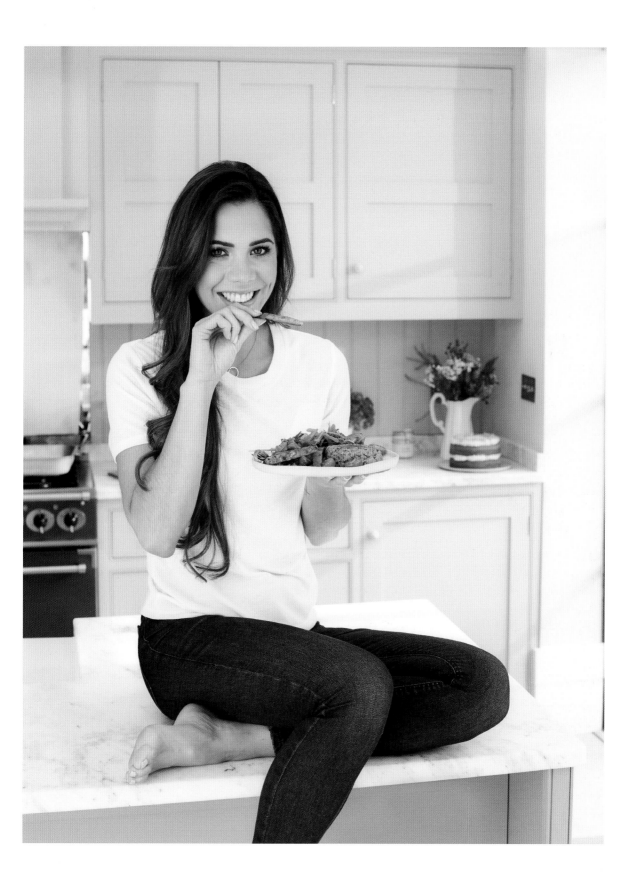

BALSAMIC BEEF BURGERS

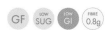

**MAKES 6 SMALL OR
4 LARGE BURGERS**

3 tbsp olive oil

1 onion, diced

1 garlic clove, grated

500g lean minced beef

2 tbsp balsamic glaze

¼ tsp salt

½ tsp pepper

2 tbsp chopped fresh
parsley or 1 tsp dried
parsley

TO SERVE (OPTIONAL)

4–6 burger buns

2 heads of romaine lettuce,
leaves separated

Pickled Red Onion
(see page 94)

4 gherkins, sliced

Slices of Cheddar or
Monterey Jack cheese

2 beef tomatoes, sliced

Salt and black pepper

*These burgers are wonderfully juicy and tender – best served piled high
with tomato, lettuce, cheese, gherkins and pickled red onion.*

Place 1 tablespoon of the olive oil in a large saucepan over a medium heat.
When hot, fry the onion and garlic for 5 minutes, until soft. Remove from
heat and set aside.

Place the beef in a large bowl with the balsamic glaze, salt, pepper,
parsley, onions and garlic. Using your hands, mix until well combined.
Divide the mixture into 4–6 equal pieces, then shape them into burgers
about 2cm thick.

Pour the remaining 2 tablespoons olive oil into the frying pan over a
medium–high heat. When hot, cook the burgers for about 5 minutes
on each side, depending on how well done you like them.

Serve with the buns and other accompaniments, if using.

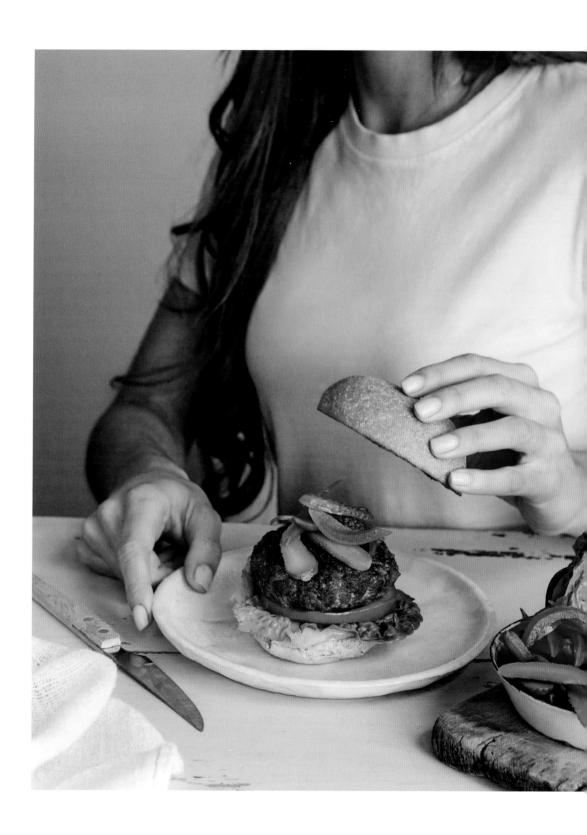

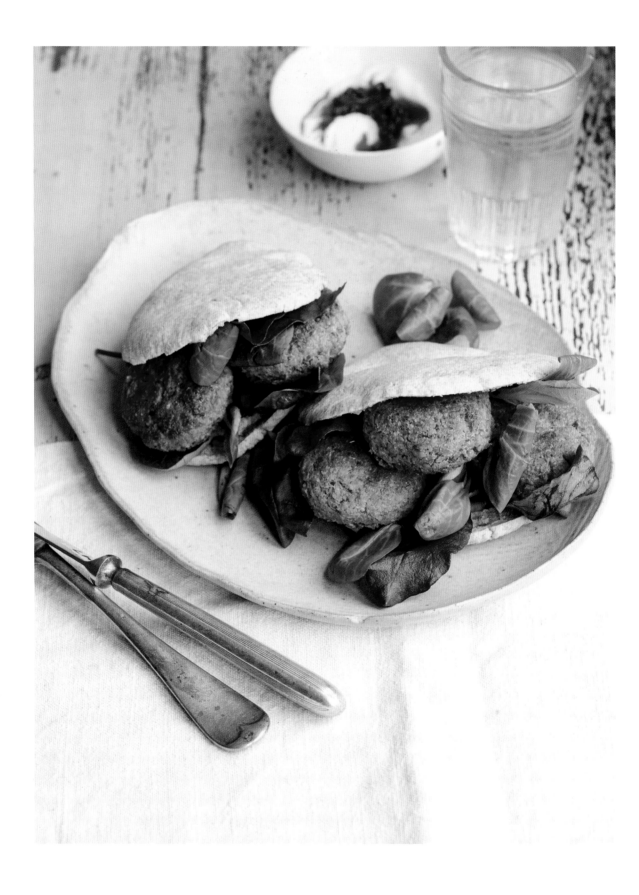

COURGETTE + HARISSA FALAFELS

MAKES 12

I love falafels in salads, in pitta bread, in wraps, and even as a snack on their own. They're high in protein and fibre, plus they're fork free, so they're the ultimate lunchbox heroes.

50g courgette, grated

3 tbsp olive oil

½ white onion, diced

1 garlic clove, chopped

1 x 400g tin of chickpeas, rinsed and drained

1 tbsp harissa paste

1 tsp tahini

50g oats

½ tsp smoked paprika

½ tsp ground cumin

1–2 tbsp spelt or wheat flour, for rolling

Salt and black pepper

TO SERVE (OPTIONAL)

Pitta breads

Green salad

Natural yogurt

Harissa paste

Preheat the oven to 180°C/350°F/gas mark 4. Line a baking tray with baking parchment.

Place the grated courgette on kitchen paper or a clean tea-towel and squeeze out the excess moisture.

Place a tablespoon of the oil in a frying pan over a medium heat. When hot, fry the onion and garlic for 3–4 minutes, until soft.

Place the courgette and chickpeas in a blender or food processor. Add the fried garlic and onion, the harissa paste, tahini, oats and spices, plus some salt and pepper. Blend until everything comes together into a dough.

Divide the dough into 12 equal pieces. Roll each piece into a ball, then roll each ball lightly in the flour.

Place a tablespoon of the remaining oil in a large non-stick frying pan over a medium–high heat. When hot, fry the falafels for 2–3 minutes under golden all over. Transfer to a lined baking tray and bake for 25 minutes.

Serve the falafels stuffed into pitta bread, hot or cold, with salad, natural yogurt and harissa paste.

If stored in an airtight container in the fridge, the falafels will keep for 2–3 days.

SWEET POTATO FALAFELS

MAKES 18–20

Make these the night before work or classes, and pack them up for lunch with some pitta bread, hummus and rocket leaves. They will keep for 2–3 days in the fridge, so you won't have to make lunch for a while.

750g sweet potatoes, peeled

2 tbsp olive oil

1 tsp ground cumin

1 tsp ground coriander

½ tsp ground cinnamon

2 garlic cloves, crushed

Small handful of flat-leaf parsley leaves, finely chopped

Small handful of coriander leaves, finely chopped

Zest of ½ lemon

4 tbsp white spelt flour

Salt and black pepper

TO SERVE

Pitta breads

Hummus

Rocket leaves

Preheat the oven to 200°C/400°F/gas mark 6. Line 2 baking trays with baking parchment.

Chop the sweet potatoes into bite-sized chunks and place them in a bowl. Add the olive oil and some salt, toss well, then transfer to a roasting tin. Roast for 25 minutes, until cooked through.

Put the cooked sweet potato into a blender or food processor and blitz to a purée. Transfer to a bowl, add the ground spices, the garlic, chopped herbs and lemon zest and mix well. Sprinkle in the spelt flour, stir through, then season to taste with salt and pepper.

Spoon heaped tablespoons of the sticky mixture onto the prepared baking trays, shaping them into slightly flattened rounds. Roast for 15–20 minutes, until they take on a bit of colour and firm up.

Serve the falafels stuffed into pitta bread with hummus and rocket, or as part of a salad.

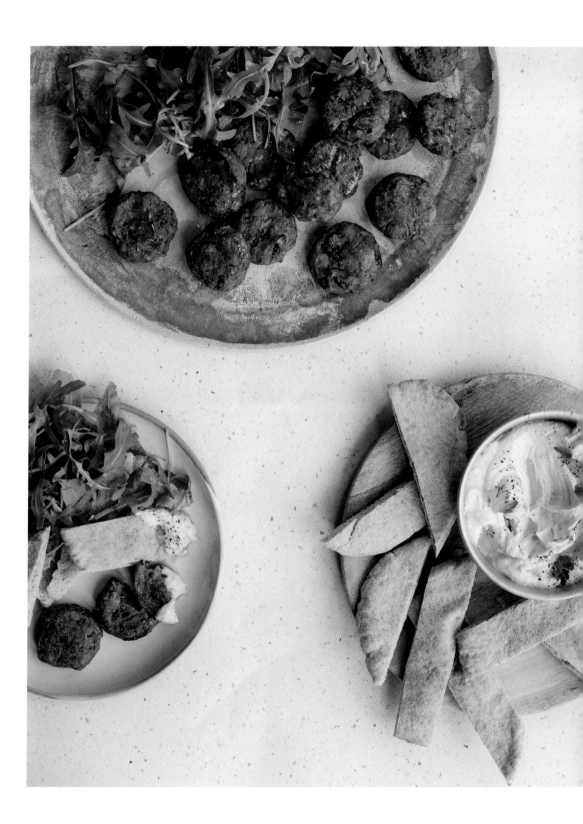

PICKLED RED ONION

MAKES 1 X 350G JAR

You either love this or hate it. I love it, and I hope you do too. I always top my burgers, falafels and tacos with a spoonful of this delicious pickle, so I get through it pretty fast. Not to worry, though – it keeps for up to a month in the fridge, and it's easy to double up the batch if you wish.

1 tbsp sugar
1 garlic clove, peeled and
   left whole
1 tsp salt
1 tsp peppercorns
250ml white wine vinegar
2–3 small onions, thinly
   sliced

Put the sugar, garlic, salt, and peppercorns in a small saucepan. Add the vinegar and stir until the sugar and salt have dissolved. Cover and bring to the boil over a medium–high heat.

Add the onion to the boiling liquid and allow to soften for 1–2 minutes.

Take the pan off the heat and use a spatula or the back of a spoon to press the onion down so all the pieces are submerged. Set aside to cool to room temperature.

Once cool, use the onions immediately or transfer them and their liquid to a lidded non-reactive container (glass, ceramic or plastic). Store in the fridge, where the pickle will keep for 3–4 weeks.

RAINBOW SLAW WITH ASIAN VINAIGRETTE

SERVES 6–8 AS A SIDE

½ head each of red and white
   cabbage, thinly sliced
2 carrots, shaved into ribbons
4 spring onions, chopped
4 tbsp olive oil
1 tbsp soy sauce
Juice of ½ lemon
1 garlic clove, grated
1 tsp sugar
2 tbsp sesame seeds
Salt

The perfect crunchy accompaniment to any burger or falafel. I hand-shred my vegetables because I like them chunky, but you can prep them in a food processor for finer slaw if you prefer.

Place the vegetables in a large salad bowl.

Put the olive oil, soy sauce, lemon juice, garlic and sugar in a bowl and whisk together. Taste and season with salt.

Pour the dressing over the vegetables and toss until well coated. Sprinkle the sesame seeds on top and serve.

WEEKDAY DINNERS

Many of us have a long commute to work, which can mean leaving the house before 6am and getting back when it's starting to get dark. How nice is the thought when you're on the way home, perhaps stuck in traffic or riding on a stuffy train, to know that you have already prepped your meal, or that you have the ingredients for a dish that will take less than 30 minutes to make? Dreamy . . . you may even have time for that bath now.

In this section you will find batch-cook recipes, such as my Chickpea Curry and Spicy Prawn Stew (see pages 96 and 99), that you can cook on a Sunday and portion out for the week, as well as super-simple meals with a handful of ingredients that you can whip up in under 30 minutes – No Fasta Pasta, for example, or my Bish-bash-bosh Chicken Tray Bake (see pages 120 and 108).

CHICKPEA, CARROT + RED PEPPER CURRY

 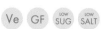

SERVES 4

I like to call this 'my little bowl of sunshine' because it's jam-packed with beautifully vibrant colours from the carrots, peppers, tomatoes and spices. These vegetables are particularly rich in carotenoids, which have been linked to multiple health benefits, especially their protective role in eye health.

1 tbsp coconut oil

1 onion, finely sliced

2 garlic cloves, grated

1 tsp garam masala

1 tsp ground turmeric

1 tsp ground cumin

¼ tsp chilli powder, or more according to preference

¼ tsp salt

1 tbsp tomato purée

1 x 400g tin of tomatoes

2 carrots, peeled and chopped

1 bell pepper (yellow, orange or red), deseeded and sliced

1 x 400ml tin of reduced-fat coconut milk

1 x 400g tin of chickpeas, drained and rinsed

TO SERVE (OPTIONAL)

Brown rice

1 large roasted sweet potato, to stuff with the curry (how I like it)

Heat the oil in a large saucepan and add the onion. Cook until softened, about 5 minutes. Add the garlic, spices, salt and tomato purée and stir to combine. Cook for 1–2 minutes.

Tip in the tomatoes, breaking them up with a wooden spoon, and simmer for 10 minutes. Add the carrots and pepper, then pour in the coconut milk and bring to the boil. Simmer for 15 minutes, until the sauce has thickened and the carrots have softened but still have a bite to them.

Add the chickpeas and warm through for a further 5 minutes.

Eat immediately, served with rice or stuffed into a baked sweet potato. Alternatively, store in an airtight container in the fridge for last-minute dinners after work.

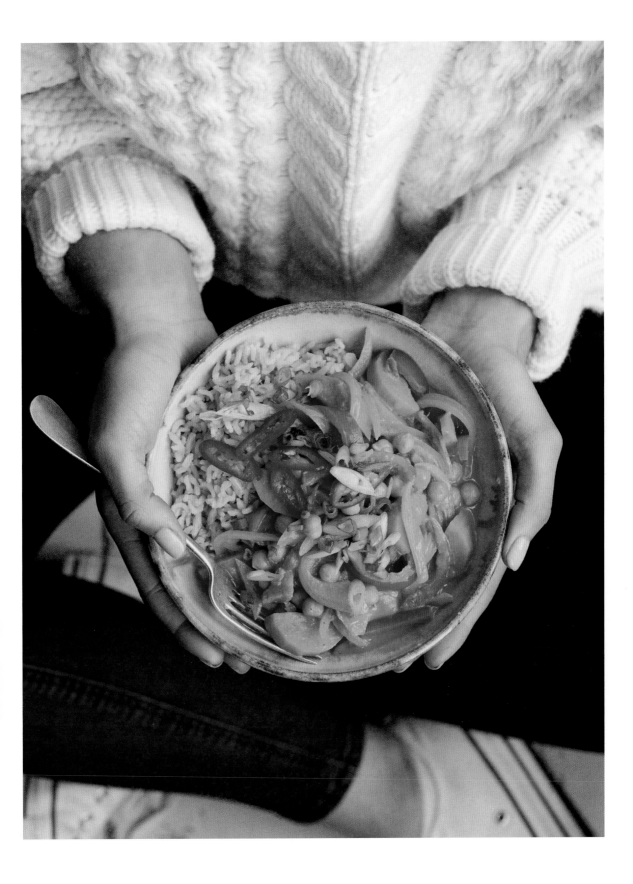

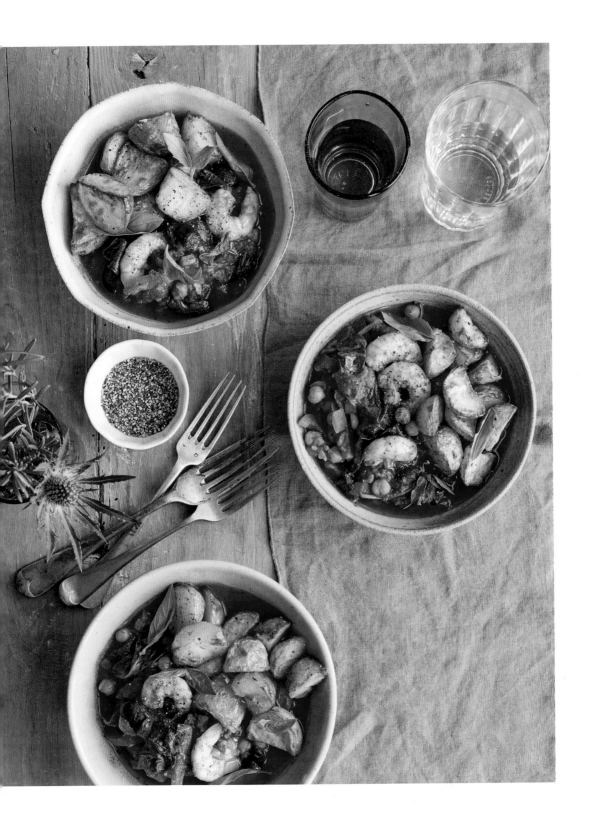

SPICY PRAWN + CHICKPEA STEW
WITH ROASTED GARLIC POTATOES

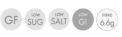

SERVES 4

1 tbsp olive oil

1 white onion, diced

2 garlic cloves, grated

1 tbsp tomato purée

2 x 400g tins of tomatoes

1 red bell pepper,
deseeded and sliced

1 tsp dried oregano

1 tsp dried basil

½ tsp salt

1 tsp brown sugar
(optional, but it does
enhance tangy tomatoes)

½ tsp chilli flakes (optional)

Handful of pitted black
olives, chopped
(optional)

4 sundried tomatoes,
chopped (optional)

1 x 400g tin of chickpeas,
drained and rinsed

300g cooked prawns,
peeled

Handful of spinach

Fresh basil, to serve
(optional)

FOR THE GARLIC
POTATOES

500g new potatoes,
quartered

1 tbsp olive oil

1 garlic clove, finely
chopped

Salt and black pepper

I made this recipe for my sister and brother-in-law and we finished all four portions between the three of us, mopping up the remaining sauce with some crusty bread. Trust me, it's seriously more-ish. It's also a great make-ahead dish for work, or to have ready in the fridge for after work. I love it served with prawns, but it would also taste amazing teamed with chicken, chorizo or butternut squash.

Preheat the oven to 220°C/425°F/gas mark 7.

First prepare the potatoes. Place them in a pan of boiling water and parboil for 7–8 minutes. Drain well, transfer to a roasting tray, then toss them with the olive oil, garlic and a little salt and pepper. Roast for 20 minutes, until crisp and golden.

Meanwhile, heat the oil in a large frying pan, then fry the onion and garlic on a low heat, stirring from time to time, until almost translucent.

Stir in the tomato purée, then add the tinned tomatoes, breaking them up with the back of a wooden spoon or a potato masher. Add the red pepper, dried herbs and salt, and the optional sugar, chilli flakes, olives and sundried tomatoes if you wish. Mix well, then simmer for about 15 minutes, stirring from time to time, until the sauce has thickened.

Once the sauce thickens, stir in chickpeas and prawns and let them warm through for just 3–5 minutes. Add the spinach and cook for a further 1–2 minutes, until the leaves have wilted.

Sprinkle with the fresh basil (if using) and serve with the roasted garlic potatoes.

SWEET POTATO, HAZELNUT + GOAT'S CHEESE SALAD IN A POMEGRANATE DRESSING

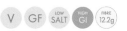

SERVES 2

This salad gives me life! It's possibly my favourite of the salad recipes I make. It's so satisfying yet light, sweet but savoury, and fresh but still warming that it can be eaten at any time of the year, or at any time of day. The toasted hazelnuts add something special to the dish, but you can use any nuts or seeds you like.

2 small sweet potatoes
   (about 350–400g
   in total)
2 tbsp olive oil
1 tbsp honey or
   maple syrup
½ red onion, sliced into
   semicircles
100g tenderstem broccoli
30g hazelnuts
100g rocket leaves
2 whole cooked beetroot
   (see tip, page 84),
   peeled and cut into
   chunks
80g goat's cheese,
   crumbled
40g pomegranate seeds
Salt

FOR THE DRESSING
1 tbsp pomegranate juice
1 tbsp balsamic vinegar
1 tsp sugar or honey
2 tbsp olive oil

Preheat the oven to 180°C/350°F/gas mark 4. Line a baking tray with baking parchment.

Chop the sweet potatoes into bite-sized chunks and spread them out in the prepared tray. Drizzle with a tablespoon of the olive oil and the honey, and sprinkle with a pinch of salt. Bake for 35 minutes, until soft and golden.

Meanwhile, heat the remaining tablespoon of oil in a frying pan and fry the onion for 1–2 minutes. Add the broccoli and continue to cook for 5–10 minutes, until it begins to soften but still has a bite to it (the time depends on the size of your broccoli stalks). Remove from the heat.

Place the hazelnuts in another baking tray and roast for 8–10 minutes, until golden and fragrant.

Meanwhile, put all the dressing ingredients into a lidded jar and shake well, or whisk in a small bowl.

Place the rocket in a large serving bowl. Add the broccoli mixture, the roasted sweet potato, beetroot and goat's cheese. Pour the dressing on top, toss together gently and sprinkle with the toasted hazelnuts and pomegranate seeds.

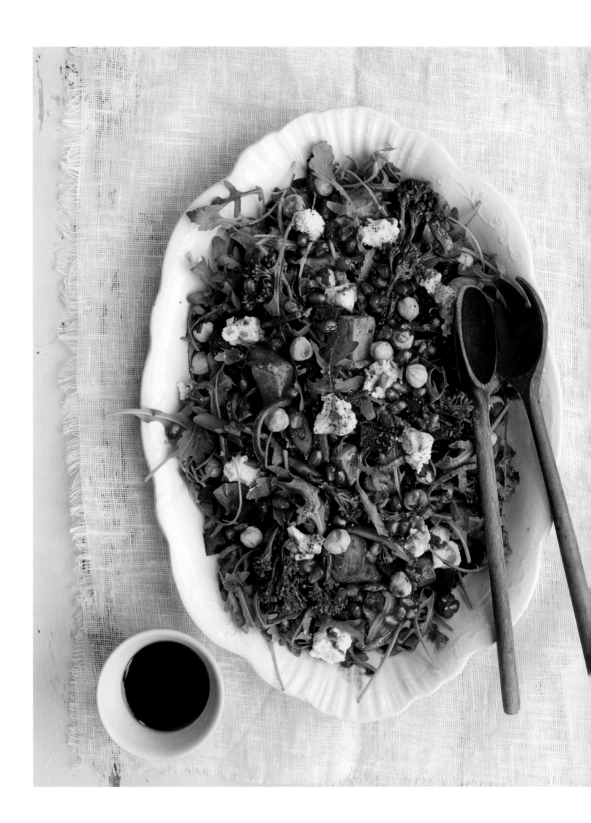

BEETROOT + COCONUT DHAL

  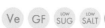

SERVES 4–6

I grew up with a group of eight friends who all lived in the same village as me, and we went to the same primary and secondary schools. We are still close friends, despite living in different countries and having taken very different directions in life. Sophie Van Dijk is one of the group and a huge foodie, just like me. She did a business degree at university, but recently left her job to study at Ballymaloe Cookery School, which is run by the renowned Darina Allen. I am so incredibly proud of Sophie and excited to share her gorgeous dhal recipe here. The beetroot gives it a wonderful pinkish-red colour, but also brings a slight sweetness to the dish.

1 x 400ml tin of full-fat coconut milk

1 tbsp coconut oil

1 heaped tsp cumin seeds

200g uncooked red lentils, rinsed and drained

1 tsp ground turmeric

1 heaped tsp garam masala

1 heaped tsp ground coriander

½ tsp chilli powder or cayenne pepper

500g cooked whole beetroot, peeled (see tip, page 84)

TO SERVE (OPTIONAL)
Boiled rice

Natural yogurt

Freshly chopped coriander

Shake the tin of coconut milk thoroughly because the water and cream sometimes separate inside it. Open the tin, as you will need it in a hurry, but set it aside for now.

Melt the coconut oil in a large saucepan over a medium heat. Add the cumin seeds and fry gently for just 15–20 seconds, until they start to smell aromatic. Add the coconut milk straight away to prevent the seeds burning.

Add the lentils and spices to the pan and stir together. Half-fill the empty coconut milk tin with water, swish it around to loosen any remaining bits, then add the liquid to the pan.

Bring the dhal to the boil, then simmer for about 15 minutes, until the lentils are tender, almost mushy and only just holding their shape.

Meanwhile, grate the beetroot coarsely. When the lentils are ready, stir in the beetroot and you're done.

This dhal is gorgeous served with rice, a dollop of natural yogurt and a sprinkling of coriander.

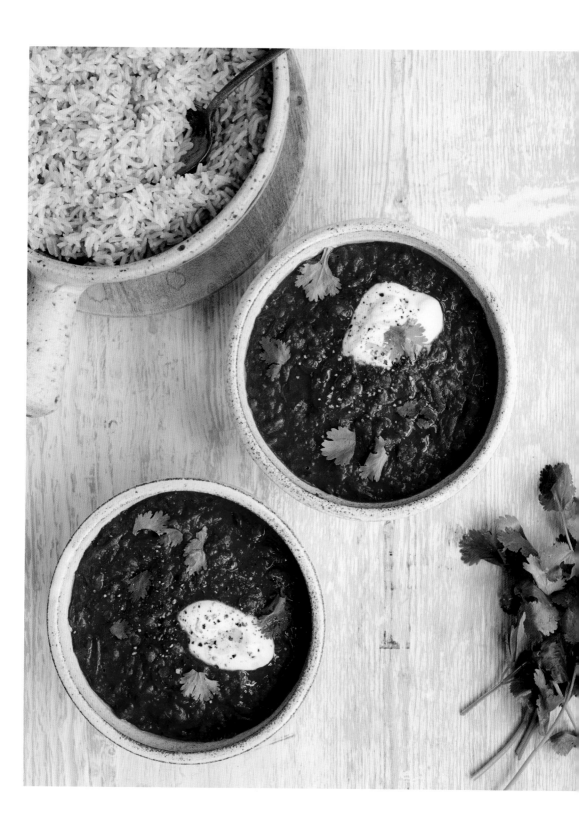

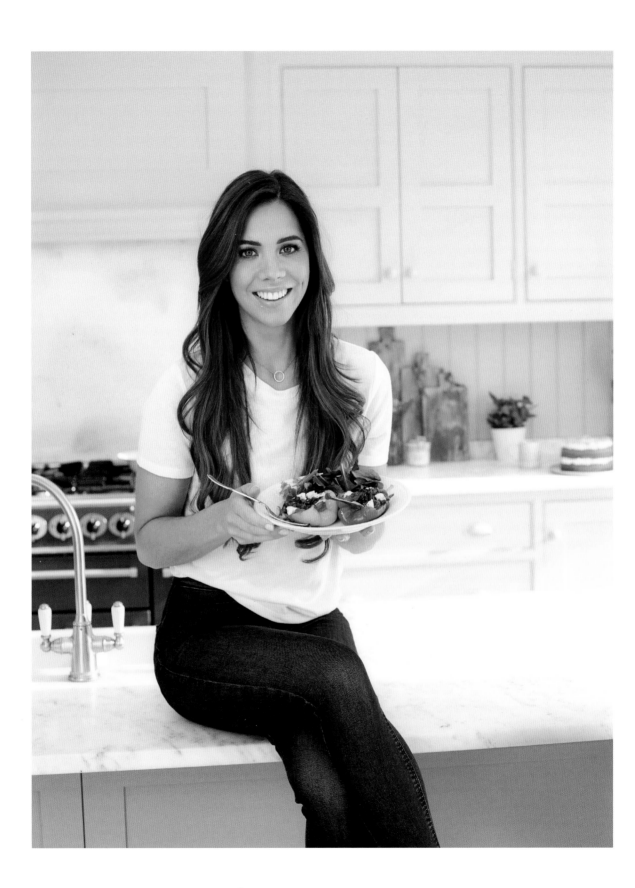

STUFFED PEPPERS WITH LENTILS + FETA

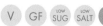

SERVES 4

This is a super-speedy recipe, which can be knocked up in half an hour if you use a packet or tin of ready-cooked lentils. If you have no feta, goat's cheese or ricotta would also taste great.

4 bell peppers, halved lengthways and deseeded

3 tbsp extra-virgin olive oil

1 red onion, finely chopped

1 garlic clove, crushed

200g cooked lentils

200g cherry tomatoes, chopped

Handful of mint leaves, finely chopped

Handful of flat-leaf parsley, finely chopped

Juice of 1 lemon

120g feta cheese (or maybe add some dollops of pesto instead)

Salt and black pepper

Green salad, to serve

Preheat the oven to 200°C/400°F/gas mark 6. Line a baking tray with tinfoil or baking parchment.

Place the peppers on the prepared tray and drizzle with 1–2 tablespoons of the olive oil. Use your hands to rub the oil all over the peppers, then arrange them cut side up and sprinkle with salt and pepper. Roast for 20–25 minutes, until tender.

Meanwhile, heat 1 tablespoon of the oil in a frying pan and fry the onions for 5 minutes. Add the garlic and continue cooking for another minute. Stir in the lentils, tomatoes, herbs and lemon juice. Season with salt and pepper.

Spoon the mixture into the peppers and crumble the feta cheese on top. Return to the oven for 5–10 minutes.

Serve the stuffed peppers with a leafy green salad.

FUSS-FREE PHO

SERVES 2

Pho (pronounced 'fuh') is a Vietnamese noodle broth, traditionally served with chicken (pho ga) or beef (pho bo). Traditional pho takes several hours to make, and not many of us have the time or patience for that, so I've devised my own recipe, which takes about half an hour in total to prepare and cook.

For a vegan/vegetarian version, omit the fish sauce and replace the chicken with a boiled egg or crispy Teriyaki Tofu (see page 110).

1 litre chicken, beef or vegetable stock

1 small onion, diced

2 garlic cloves, finely chopped

5cm piece of fresh root ginger, peeled and thinly sliced

1 tsp Chinese five spice

2 tbsp soy sauce

1 tbsp fish sauce

150g mangetout or baby corn or tenderstem broccoli, or a mixture

50g beansprouts

2 nests of rice noodles

200g cooked chicken, shredded

2 spring onions, sliced

1 red chilli, sliced

Handful of fresh herbs (e.g. basil, mint and coriander)

Lime wedges

Pour the stock into a large saucepan and add the onion, garlic, ginger, Chinese five spice, soy sauce and fish sauce. Bring to the boil, then cover and simmer for 15 minutes.

Add the vegetables and beansprouts to the pan and cook until softened, a further 3–5 minutes.

Place each nest of noodles in a shallow bowl. Ladle the stock and veg on top of them.

Top with the chicken, spring onions, chilli, fresh herbs and lime wedges.

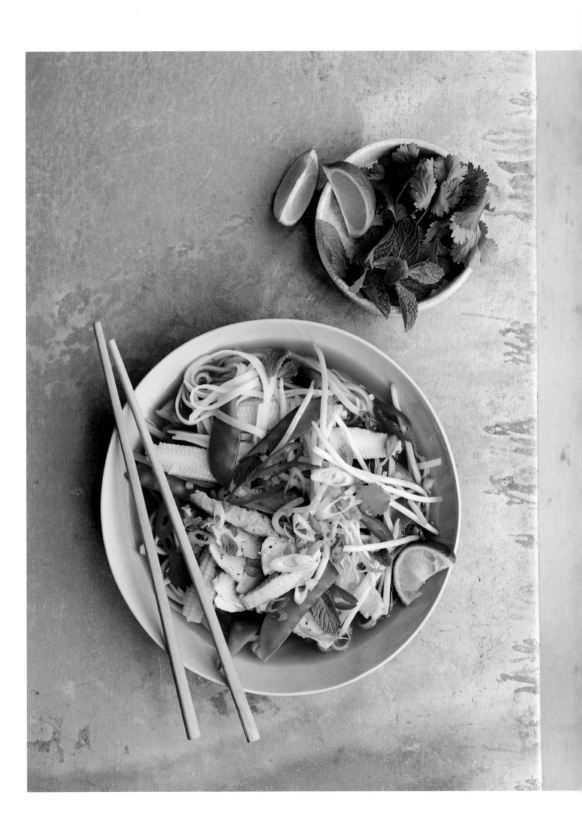

BISH-BASH-BOSH CHICKEN TRAY BAKE WITH LENTILS + ROASTED VEGETABLES

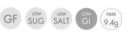

SERVES 4

As the name suggests, this is one of those meals that requires simple ingredients, one pan and little kitchen experience. Just remember to marinate things the night before for full-on flavour the next day.

4 skinless chicken breasts, chopped into large chunks

2 bell peppers, deseeded and sliced

1 courgette, sliced

1 red onion, cut into thin wedges

4 whole garlic cloves, peeled and used whole

Olive oil, to drizzle

400–500g cooked Puy lentils

Salt and black pepper

FOR THE MARINADE

2 tbsp harissa paste

1 tbsp olive oil

1 tbsp honey or maple syrup

Juice and zest of ½ lemon

First make the marinade. Place the ingredients for it in a large bowl and stir together. Add the chicken pieces and rub the marinade into them thoroughly. Cover and leave in the fridge overnight, or for at least 1–2 hours.

Preheat the oven to 180°C/350°F/gas mark 4.

Place the vegetables and garlic in a roasting tray, drizzle with olive oil and season with salt and pepper. Add the chicken and its marinade, mix together and cook in the oven for 20–25 minutes, until the juices run clear.

Add the lentils, stirring to combine. Return to the oven for a further 5–10 minutes, until the chicken is cooked through and the vegetables are tender.

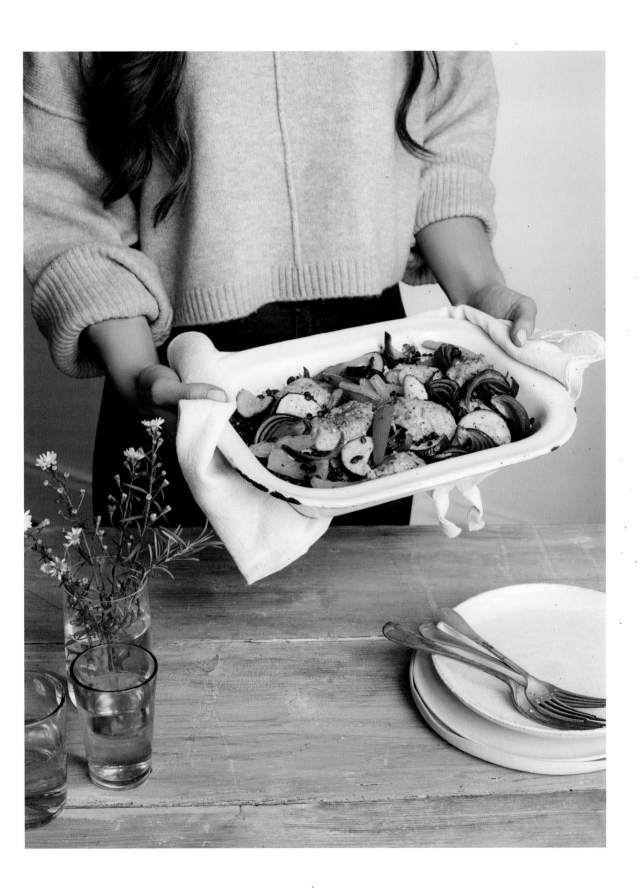

TERIYAKI TOFU STIR-FRY

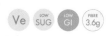

SERVES 2

Tofu is one of those foods that can taste horrible if it's not cooked well, so here are a few keys to making it deliciously crisp. First of all, choose firm or extra-firm tofu. The next step is to squeeze out as much moisture as possible by wrapping it in kitchen paper or a cloth, putting it in a colander set over a bowl, and placing a weight on top for an hour or two. After that, I like to marinate it lightly, for about an hour, to infuse flavour without it going soggy. Finally, you can bake the tofu at 180°C/350°F/gas mark 4 for 30–40 minutes, or, what I like to do, fry it in a hot pan for 10 minutes.

3 tbsp soy sauce

2 tbsp mirin

200g extra-firm tofu, drained (see introduction)

2 tbsp coconut oil

1 garlic clove, grated

½ red chilli, deseeded and finely sliced (optional)

5cm piece of fresh root ginger, peeled and finely sliced

100g mixed mushrooms, sliced

4 spring onions, sliced at an angle

2 heads of pak choi, leaves separated

Handful of peanuts, roughly chopped

200g cooked rice, to serve

To make a marinade, place 2 tablespoons of the soy sauce in a small bowl, add the mirin and whisk together.

Chop the tofu into bite-sized pieces and place in a shallow dish. Pour the marinade over the tofu, cover and leave to marinate in the fridge for 1 hour.

Put 1 tablespoon of the coconut oil in a wok or frying pan over a medium–high heat. When hot, add the tofu and its marinade and fry for 5–10 minutes, stirring every 1–2 minutes, until the tofu is golden and crisp.

Add the garlic, chilli, ginger, mushrooms and spring onions and stir-fry for a further 2–3 minutes.

Add the pak choi and the remaining tablespoon of soy sauce and fry for another minute or so, until the leaves have started to wilt slightly.

Sprinkle with the peanuts and serve immediately with the rice.

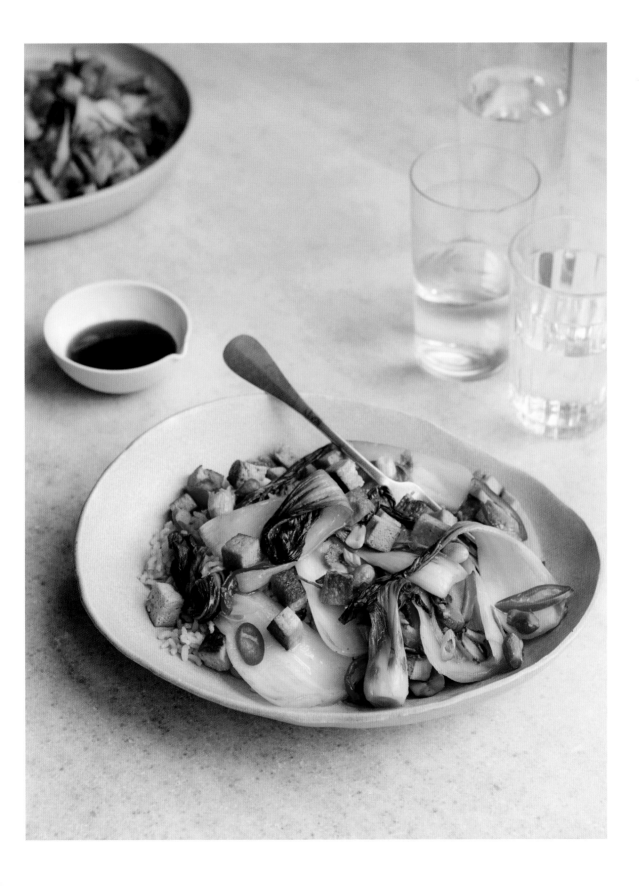

FIBRE + GUT HEALTH

The human gut is home to trillions of bacteria, known as the gut microbiota. We are conditioned to view bacteria as a bad thing, but some actually offer many benefits – particularly the good guys in the gut.

Healthy gut bacteria have multiple roles, which include discouraging the growth of disease-causing bacteria, producing vitamins and chemicals, aiding the absorption of nutrients and helping the body to digest fibre.

Each human being has a set of microbes as unique as a fingerprint. Those microbes are influenced by where and how you were born, your genes, environment, diet and even your life experiences. In recent years, scientists have become more and more interested in the microbiota as they've come to realise just how important it is, not only for the digestive system, but for the entire body, from the brain and skin to the immune system. This community of bacteria may be the driving force behind your mood, appetite, weight and so much more. But you can influence your gut microbiota, just as it influences you – for better and for worse – through food, medication, sleep and environment.

HOW TO HELP YOUR GUT MICROBIOTA TO THRIVE

There are several pretty easy things you can do to ensure the good health of your gut.

EAT A VARIETY OF FOODS

As a general rule, the more diverse your diet, the more diverse and healthy your gut microbiota will be. There are between 250,000 and 300,000 known edible plant species, but despite this, 75% of the world's food comes from only twelve plant species and five animal species. Be a rebel this week and add a fruit, vegetable, grain or legume that you've never tried before to your shopping basket.

EAT MORE FIBRE

Adults should be aiming to consume around 30g of fibre a day, but most of us massively undershoot that. The western diet is heavily based on refined foods, such as white bread, pasta, rice, cakes and sweets, which are stripped of their fibre (along with vitamins and minerals) during processing. While this might make them easier to digest, it means they don't offer much nourishment to our little friends in the gut. If you're not accustomed to having much fibre in your diet, increase your daily intake slowly, by just 2–3g (about the amount of fibre in an apple) and see how you feel. Some people can be very sensitive to increases in fibre and may find that they experience some bloating and wind.

EAT PROBIOTIC-RICH FOODS

Probiotics are live beneficial bacteria that occur naturally in most fermented foods, such as kimchi, sauerkraut, kefir (a fermented milk drink) and kombucha (fermented sweet tea).

EAT PREBIOTIC-RICH FOODS

Prebiotics are a source of food for probiotics to grow, multiply, survive and thrive in the gut. They essentially act as the fertiliser for your gut garden of microbes. Prebiotics are typically soluble fibres found in foods such as artichokes, onions, garlic, chicory, asparagus and leeks.

SHOULD YOU TAKE A PROBIOTIC SUPPLEMENT?

Currently, there is no convincing evidence to suggest that healthy people will benefit from taking a probiotic supplement.

REDUCE THE AMOUNT OF SUGARS + SWEETENERS IN YOUR DIET

Sugar alcohols, such as xylitol and erythritol, are used as substitutes for sugar in low-calorie and low-sugar food and drink. They contain fewer calories than table sugar and natural sweeteners such as honey, so are often used in so-called 'diet' foods. Recent evidence from mice studies demonstrated that ingesting some types of artificial sweeteners might lead to obesity and type 2 diabetes by disrupting the gut microbiota. These sweeteners are also difficult to digest, and fermentation of these substances by gut bacteria may lead to wind, bloating and diarrhoea.

AVOID UNNECESSARY ANTIBIOTICS, PAINKILLERS + SUPPLEMENTS

Antibiotics can wipe out both good and bad bacteria, so it's important to nourish your gut microbiota with prebiotic- and probiotic-rich foods following a course of antibiotics, and also to avoid taking them unless advised to do so by your doctor. I often come across patients who have picked up antibiotics abroad, or have some left over at home from the last time they were unwell, and they use them to self-medicate if feeling under the weather. The thing is, antibiotics don't work for viral infections, such as coughs and colds, or the flu; and many mild bacterial infections often get better on their own without antibiotics. Taking these drugs unnecessarily won't make you better any quicker, and you'll have wiped out your gut microbes into the bargain.

TAKE TIME TO BREATHE + UNWIND

It's well established in scientific literature that bacteria in the gut affect our brain function, stress levels and mood. In turn, our stress levels can also have a profound effect on our gut microbiota. Whether it's mindfulness and meditation that helps you unwind, or something as simple as going for a ten-minute walk, my prescription is – do it!

WHISTLE-STOP TOUR THROUGH IBS

Irritable bowel syndrome, or IBS, is a common condition affecting the gut, and diagnosed by the presence of intermittent tummy pain associated with diarrhoea, constipation, or alternating episodes of both. All these symptoms can also occur in people who have more serious conditions that can mimic IBS, such as inflammatory bowel disease and coeliac disease. It is therefore important to see your GP to have these conditions excluded before doing anything else.

WHAT CAUSES IBS?

We don't always know the cause of IBS; so the best thing is to keep a food diary to figure out the cause. It can be down to a number of things, from medication and travel to stress and diet. The main food and drink culprits seem to be alcohol, fizzy drinks, caffeine, spicy food, fatty or fried food and, in some cases, components of dairy, such as lactose.

WHAT ARE THE BEST TREATMENTS?

There is no cure for IBS, but the symptoms can often be managed through diet and lifestyle. If cutting out trigger foods identified via your food diary doesn't calm your stomach, the next is the low-FODMAP diet. FODMAP stands for fermentable oligosaccharides, disaccharides, monosaccharides and polyols, a group of carbohydrates that cannot be easily broken down or absorbed by the digestive system. It is a very restrictive diet, designed to be used only in the short term and under the guidance of a registered dietitian or nutritionist.

In some cases, medication, such as antispasmodics to relax the gut, or laxatives or anti-diarrhoeal treatments, are used to manage this condition.

The next line of management, is psychological treatment, such as mindfulness. The gut is lined with millions of nerve cells that pass messages from the gut to the brain and vice versa, so it's no surprise that what goes on within the gut may be influenced by what goes on in the head. The good news is that you don't have to wait for your doctor to refer you for treatment because mindfulness and other forms of stress management are something we can all do – and should be doing – at home.

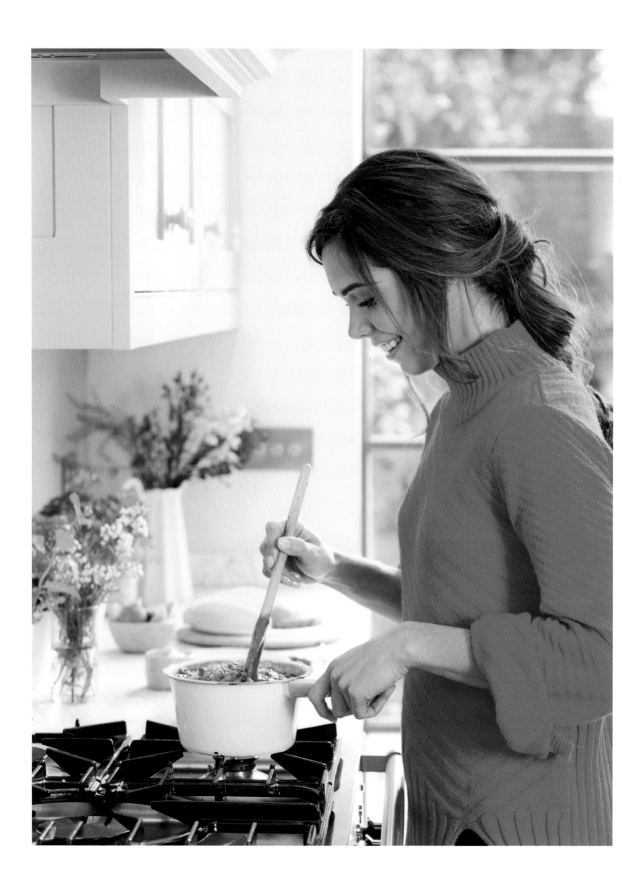

LENTIL + KIDNEY BEAN CHILLI

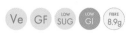

SERVES 4–6

This is so simple to make and feeds a crowd, which is why I love it on an evening when I have friends round but not much time to faff in the kitchen. For any meat-eaters reading this, you can swap the lentils for 500g lean minced beef, but don't knock the veggie version until you've tried it – you might surprise yourself.

1 tbsp olive oil

1 red onion, finely chopped

3 garlic cloves, grated

1½ tsp ground cumin

1 tsp chilli powder

1 tsp smoked paprika

2 x 400g tins of chopped tomatoes

1 bell pepper, deseeded and diced

1 vegetable stock cube, crushed

400g cooked lentils

1 x 400g tin of kidney beans, drained and rinsed

Salt and black pepper

TO SERVE

12 taco shells (100% corn tortillas), warmed

Natural yogurt, soured cream or coconut yogurt

Avocado slices

Tomato salsa, shop-bought or homemade (see page 86)

Lime wedges

Heat the oil in a large saucepan, then add the onion, garlic and spices and fry for about 5 minutes, or until the onions are soft.

Stir in the tomatoes, diced pepper, stock cube and lentils and simmer for 10 minutes, until thickened.

Add the kidney beans and heat through. Season to taste with salt and pepper.

Serve the chilli spooned into the warm taco shells, topping it with a dollop of yogurt, slices of avocado, some salsa and a squeeze of lime.

VARIATIONS: *Serve on thin slices of roasted sweet potato 'nachos', or with fluffy white rice. For a lower carbohydrate accompaniment than tacos, serve with cauliflower riced in a food processor and sautéed in a pan with some oil and a pinch of salt.*

TOMATO + PESTO COD PARCELS WITH BUTTERY GARLIC POTATOES + BROCCOLI

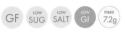

SERVES 2

This is the dinner to have after one of those crazy work days when you need something quick, easy and tasty when you get home. Don't let on I said this, but it goes really well with a small glass of Pinot Grigio.

2 cod fillets

2 tbsp pesto, shop-bought or homemade (see page 128)

10 cherry tomatoes, halved

1 lemon, halved

8–10 baby potatoes

1 tbsp butter

1 garlic clove, grated

150g tenderstem broccoli

Salt and black pepper

Preheat the oven to 180°C/350°F/gas mark 4.

Place each cod fillet on a piece of tinfoil large enough to wrap around it. Top each fillet with a tablespoon of the pesto. Sprinkle with the tomatoes, then squeeze over the juice of half the lemon. Fold the foil around the fish to seal tightly. Transfer to a roasting tin and place in the oven for 15–20 minutes, until the fish is cooked through and flakes easily.

Meanwhile, cook the potatoes in a pan of boiling water for 10–12 minutes, or until just tender. Drain well, return to the pan and add the butter, garlic and a little salt and pepper. Toss to coat the potatoes.

Steam the broccoli or simply boil it for 3–4 minutes, until tender but still with a bite. Drain, then squeeze the remaining lemon half over it.

Serve each cod parcel with the buttery garlic potatoes and the broccoli.

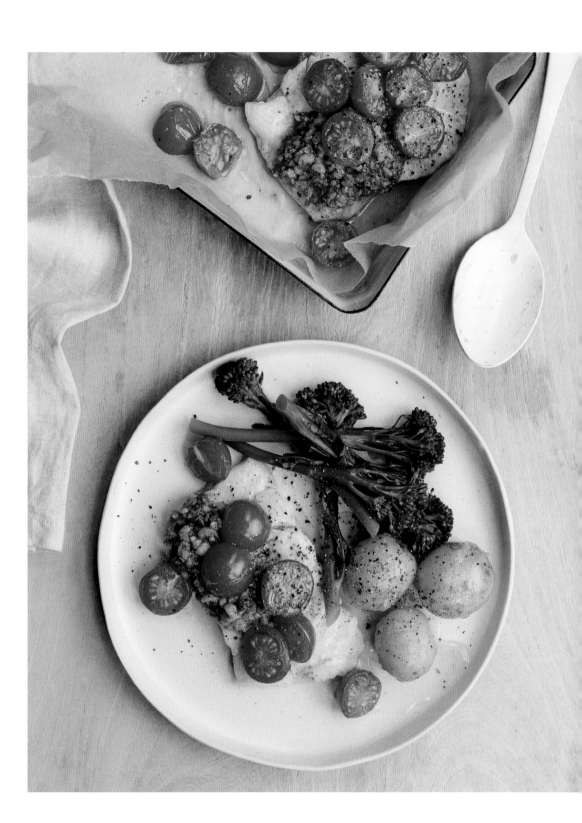

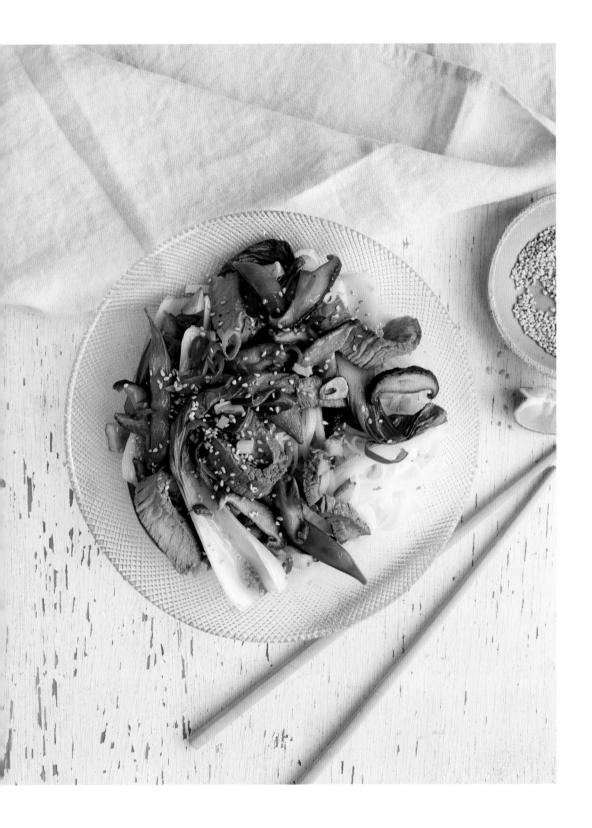

SESAME STEAK STIR-FRY WITH PAK CHOI

SERVES 4

I don't eat red meat very often, but when I do, I like to get it from the butcher so that I can choose my cut and know exactly where it has come from. For a vegan/vegetarian version of this recipe, replace the steaks with tofu or tempeh.

2–3 tbsp coconut oil
   or rapeseed oil

2 beef rump steaks

125g shiitake mushrooms,
   sliced

2 garlic cloves, sliced

1 fresh red chilli, deseeded
   and sliced

100g sugarsnap peas

200g pak choi, leaves
   separated

3 tbsp soy sauce

1 tbsp mirin

1 tsp sesame oil

4 spring onions, sliced

2 tbsp sesame seeds

Rice noodles, to serve

1 lime, cut into wedges

Place 1 tablespoon of the oil in a large wok or frying pan over a medium heat. When hot, cook the steaks for about 2 minutes on each side to serve them medium-rare. Set aside.

Add another tablespoon of the oil to the wok. When hot, fry the mushrooms, garlic and chilli for 2–3 minutes, until tender. Add the sugarsnaps and pak choi and fry for a further 1–2 minutes.

Put the soy sauce, mirin and sesame oil into a small bowl and whisk together. Pour into the wok and toss everything together.

Slice the beef into thin strips, add them to the pan and stir to combine.

Sprinkle with the spring onions and sesame seeds and serve with rice noodles and lime wedges. (A squeeze of lime really finishes this off nicely!)

NO FASTA PASTA

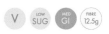

SERVES 2

Pasta with tomato sauce is one of life's simple pleasures. It's cheap, quick and tasty, and most people love it. Although it's easy to pick up a jar of pasta sauce in the supermarket, it's actually pretty easy to make your own from scratch – plus you're cutting down on the salt and sugar content found in ready-made versions.

Although delicious on its own, this pasta sauce is so versatile that you can add whatever extra ingredients you fancy. I've included some of my favourite variations on the opposite page.

PS Did you know that tinned tomatoes count towards your five-a-day?

1 tbsp olive oil

1 onion, diced

2 garlic cloves, grated

1 tbsp tomato purée

½ tsp dried basil

½ tsp dried oregano

1 x 400g tin of chopped tomatoes

½ vegetable stock cube, crumbled

½ tbsp balsamic vinegar (optional)

Handful of fresh basil leaves, chopped

150g spelt pasta

Salt and black pepper

Freshly grated Parmesan cheese (optional), to serve

Heat the oil in a large saucepan over medium heat. When hot, add the onion and garlic and cook for 3–4 minutes, until softened, stirring often.

Add the tomato purée and dried herbs and cook for 1–2 minutes, stirring constantly.

Add the tomatoes, stock cube and vinegar (if using). Season with salt and pepper, and continue cooking gently for about 15 minutes, until thickened, stirring occasionally. Turn the heat right down and add most of the fresh basil.

While the flavour of the sauce deepens, cook the pasta according to the packet instructions until al dente. Drain well, then return the pasta to the saucepan.

Mix the tomato sauce through the pasta, or serve it on top, sprinkling it with the reserved fresh basil leaves and the Parmesan.

WITH MEDITERRANEAN ROASTED VEGETABLES

Halve and deseed 2 bell peppers (1 red, 1 yellow). Cut 1 courgette into quarters, then chop into 2.5cm pieces. Peel 1 red onion and cut into 8 wedges. Preheat the oven to 200°C/400°F/gas mark 6. Place the vegetables in a large roasting tin, toss in 1 tablespoon olive oil, then roast for 30–35 minutes, or until the peppers begin to char. Serve with the pasta.

WITH GARLIC PRAWNS

Heat 1 tablespoon olive oil in a frying pan. Add 1 grated garlic clove plus 12 large, raw king prawns and fry for 4–5 minutes, until the prawns are pink and cooked through. Season with salt and pepper. Serve with the pasta.

WITH CHERRY TOMATOES AND CHILLI

Place 1 tablespoon olive oil in a frying pan over a medium heat. When hot, add 1 finely sliced garlic clove and 1 deseeded and chopped chilli. Fry for 1–2 minutes, then add 100g halved cherry tomatoes (ideally various colours). Cook for about 5 minutes, until the tomatoes begin to collapse. Serve with the pasta.

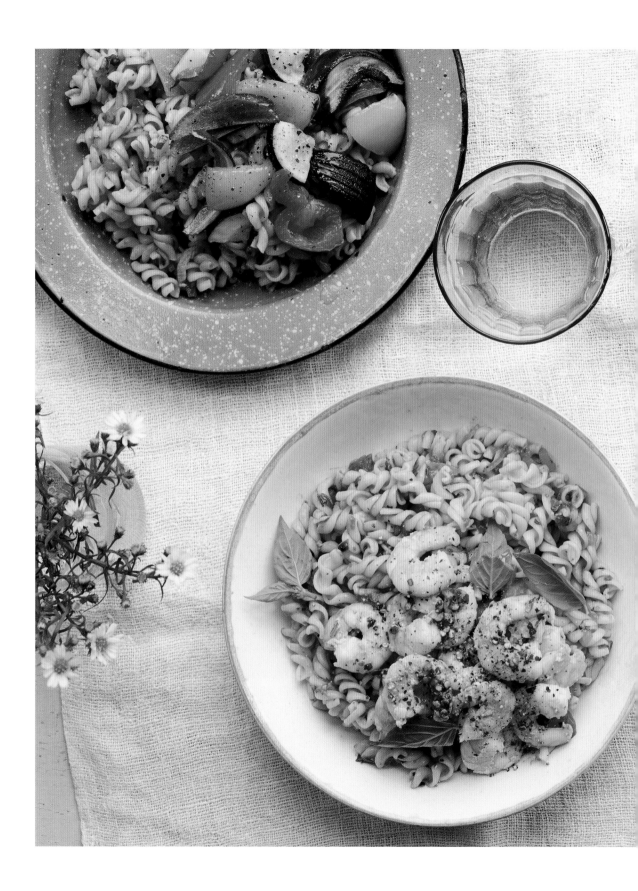

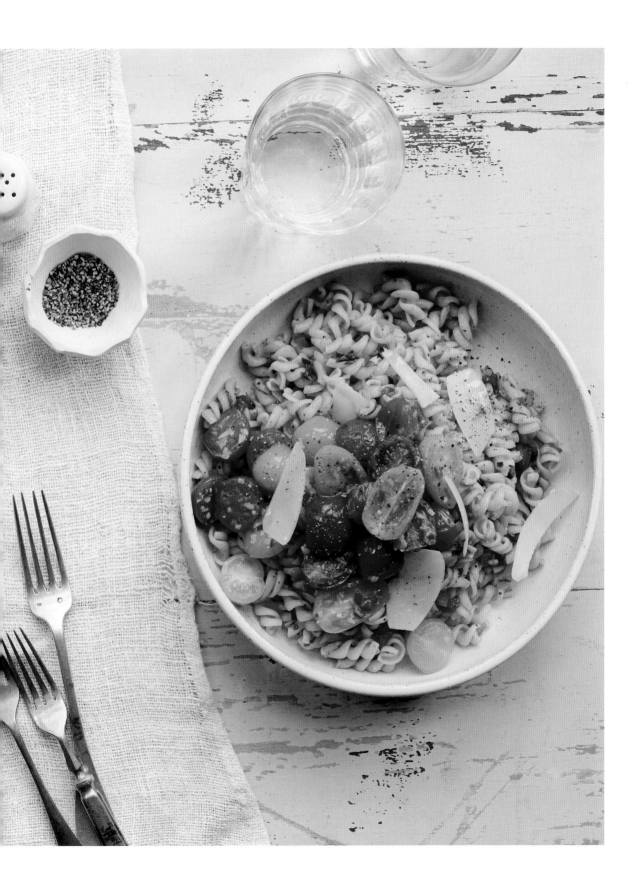

GOAT'S CHEESE + ROASTED VEGETABLE SALAD

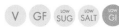

SERVES 2

This recipe requires minimal planning, preparation or cleaning up, which is why I love it. The warm vegetables and goat's cheese taste incredible together, and are just as good the next day, so make sure to double up on portions and spoon the rest into a plastic box for lunch al desko.

1 courgette, quartered lengthways then sliced widthways

1 red onion, cut into wedges

1 red bell pepper, deseeded and chopped

250g butternut squash, peeled and cubed

2 tbsp olive oil

1 tsp dried basil

1 tbsp balsamic vinegar

1 x 120g bag of rocket or baby spinach leaves

80g goat's cheese, crumbled

Salt and black pepper

Preheat the oven to 200°C/400°F/gas mark 6.

Place the vegetables in a roasting tin. Drizzle with 1 tablespoon of the olive oil, sprinkle with the basil and toss together. Roast for 25–30 minutes, until vegetables are tender and browned.

Put the balsamic vinegar and remaining tablespoon olive oil in a small bowl. Whisk together, then season with salt and pepper.

Place the rocket in a salad bowl. Add the roasted vegetables, drizzle with the dressing and toss well. Sprinkle the goat's cheese on top and serve.

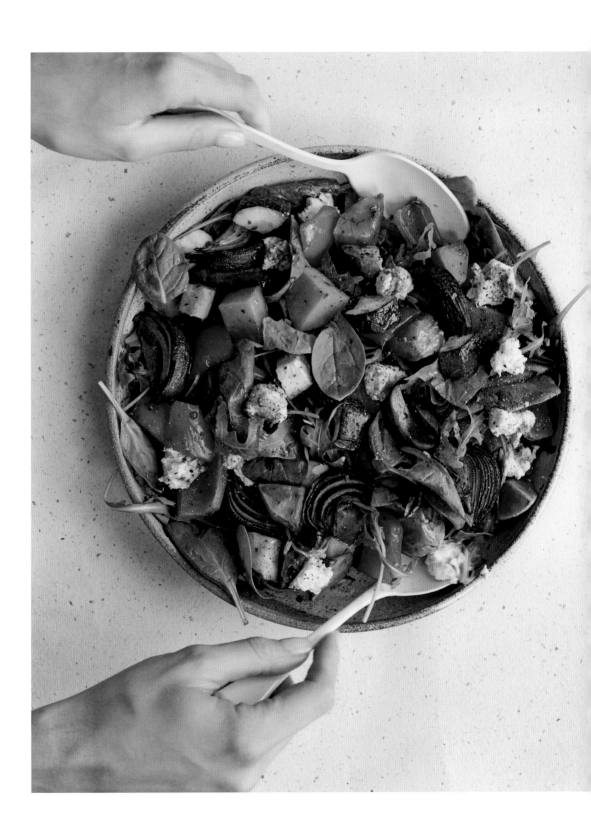

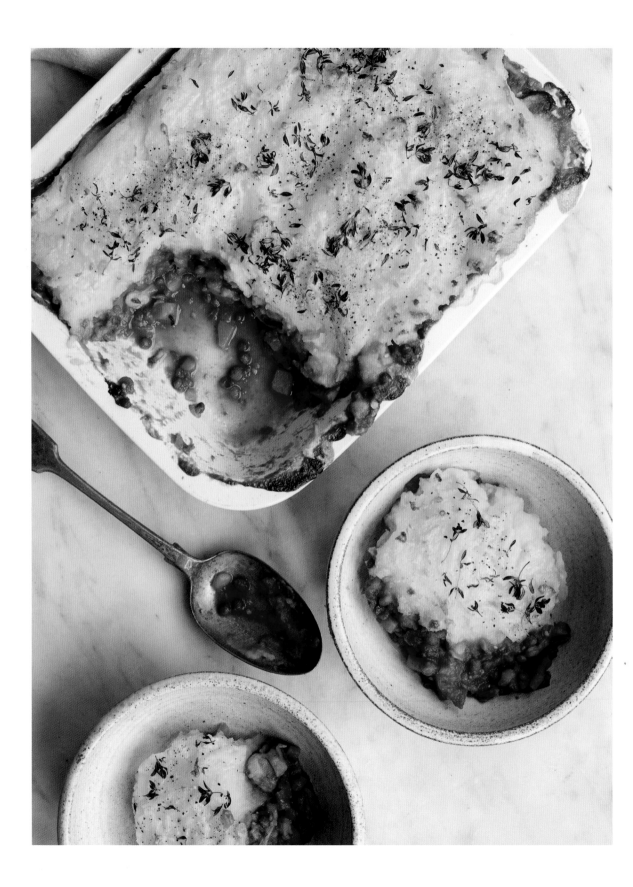

LENTIL SHEPHERD'S PIE

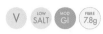

SERVES 6–8

I'm not going to lie and say that I loved shepherd's pie when growing up, because I didn't. As you probably know, the pie is traditionally made with minced lamb, but I had a pet lamb called Fluffy (a present from my uncle, who was a farmer), so I couldn't bring myself to eat the meat. Although I rarely eat lamb now, I've sort of overcome my moral dilemma. This pie is meat-free, but still packed with flavour and protein from the legumes. You can of course make it with lamb or beef mince, or do half veggie, half meat. It takes about 30–40 minutes to make, so sort of breaks my half hour rule, but you can make it the night before and heat it up after work if you're having an exceptionally busy week.

2 tbsp olive oil

2 onions, chopped

2 carrots, peeled and diced

200g button mushrooms

4 garlic cloves, crushed

1½ tsp ground cumin

2 tbsp tamari or dark
   soy sauce

1 x 400g tin of chopped
   tomatoes

2 x 400g tins of green or
   brown lentils, drained,
   or 500g cooked lentils

1 tsp fresh thyme leaves,
   to sprinkle

Freshly grated Parmesan
   cheese (optional)

FOR THE TOPPING

700g potatoes

3 tbsp butter or extra-
   virgin olive oil

Salt and black pepper

Preheat the oven to 200°C/400°F/gas mark 6. Set out a 26 x 20cm pie dish.

First make the topping. Peel and chop the potatoes and add to a pan of cold salted water. Bring to the boil, then simmer for about 10 minutes, until tender. Drain the potatoes, transfer to a bowl and mash with the butter or oil. Season to taste with salt and pepper.

While the potatoes are cooking, start the filling. Put the oil in a large frying pan over a medium–high heat. When hot, add the onions, carrots and mushrooms and sauté for 10 minutes, stirring frequently, until the onions are soft and translucent and the mushrooms are golden. Add the garlic and cumin and fry for another 2 minutes, until aromatic.

Add the tamari, tomatoes and lentils, bring to the boil, then simmer for 5 minutes. Season to taste, bearing in mind that the tamari will have provided quite a bit of salt.

Ladle the lentil mixture into the pie dish. Spread the mash over the top and smooth it out. Sprinkle with the thyme and some Parmesan (if using), then bake for 15 minutes or until golden.

HEY PRESTO, HOMEMADE PESTO

SERVES 4

Shop-bought pesto is the simplest option when you're short of time, but it's easy to make your own. Try it and you'll notice a lovely difference in flavour and texture.

1 garlic clove, peeled

2 tbsp olive oil

2 tbsp grated
  Parmesan cheese

Handful of pine nuts

Handful of fresh
  basil leaves

Salt and black pepper

Place all the ingredients in a blender and blitz to a paste that is not completely smooth. Hey presto! . . . homemade pesto.

ENERGY BOOSTS

At university I used to think bags of jelly sweets were the best source of energy when I was spending a day in the library revising for my exams. How wrong I was! Maybe they fit the bill if you're running a marathon, but that energy hit if you're sitting at your desk all day is not going to offer you any nutritional value.

In this chapter you will find fork-free snacks, such as my Hazelnutter Balls (see page 140), which you can pack up to have with your mid-morning coffee, or my Smoky Sundried Tomato + Lentil Dip with Oatcakes (see pages 131 and 215) for those days when you're stuck in work a little later than expected and you need something to keep you going until dinner time.

BAKED AUBERGINE HUMMUS

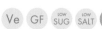

SERVES 4

1 aubergine, halved
   lengthways
1 x 400g tin of chickpeas,
   drained and rinsed
3 tbsp tahini
1 tbsp olive oil
¼ tsp salt
1 tsp smoked paprika
3 garlic cloves, peeled
Bunch of fresh parsley
Juice of 1 lemon
Black pepper

If you aren't a big aubergine lover, this may be your gateway recipe. It's creamy, garlicky and has a hint of spice that takes it to a whole new level. Roasted aubergine also gives classic hummus a lovely smoky flavour, and the addition of parsley ties this whole dip together. I really like to include some in my lunchbox.

Flick to page 215 for my super-easy Oatcakes, which are the perfect partners for this (or any) dip.

Preheat the oven to 200°C/400°F/gas mark 6. Line a baking tray with baking parchment.

Place the aubergine halves flesh-side down in the prepared baking tray and roast until soft and tender, about 35 minutes. Set aside to cool slightly.

Scoop out the aubergine flesh and place in a blender or food processor. Add the rest of the ingredients and blend until smooth and well combined. Taste and adjust the seasonings as necessary. If the mixture is too thick, add a dash of water.

Store in an airtight container in the fridge for up to 7 days.

BEETROOT, MINT + TAHINI DIP

SERVES 4

4 cooked beetroot, peeled
   (see tip, page 84)
4 tbsp tahini
2 garlic cloves, chopped
Handful of fresh mint leaves
2 tbsp extra-virgin olive oil
Juice ½ lemon

This dip is so incredibly vibrant, I love it! I've also found that it goes with virtually everything – falafel, burgers, wraps, flatbreads, salads . . . you name it. It's great for lunchboxes too, with some crunchy radishes and carrot sticks.

Put all the ingredients in a blender or food processor and blitz until smooth. If it's too thick, add a little more olive oil or lemon juice.

SMOKY SUNDRIED TOMATO + LENTIL DIP

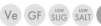 Ve GF LOW SUG LOW SALT LOW GI FIBRE 25.9g

SERVES 4

1 tbsp olive oil

1 onion, chopped

1 garlic clove, grated

1 x 400g tin of lentils, drained, or 250g cooked lentils

5 sundried tomatoes

2 tbsp tahini

1 tbsp water

Juice of 1 lemon

1 tsp smoked paprika

½ tsp ground cumin

Salt and black pepper

I made this dip as a last-minute thought when I was hosting a dinner party, and it may have been the star of the whole show. Everyone loved it as a side to their meal, and afterwards we ate the leftovers with some fresh sourdough bread and cheese.

Place the olive oil in a frying pan over a medium heat. When hot, fry the onion and garlic for 3–5 minutes, until soft. Allow to cool for 10 minutes before transferring to a blender or food processor.

Add the rest of the ingredients (apart from the seasoning) and blend until smooth and creamy. Add a tablespoon of water if the dip is too thick. Season to taste with salt and pepper.

ARTICHOKE + SPINACH DIP

 Ve GF LOW SUG LOW SALT LOW GI FIBRE 6.1g

SERVES 4

285g preserved artichoke hearts

1 garlic clove, peeled

2 handfuls of spinach

Zest and juice of 1 lemon

2 tbsp extra-virgin olive oil

2 tbsp pine nuts

Salt and black pepper

This is the ultimate Friday night dip to serve with oatcakes or crudités. I also love it on rye bread topped with smoked salmon.

Place all the ingredients (apart from the seasoning) in a blender or food processor and blitz until combined but still with a bit of texture. Season with salt and pepper.

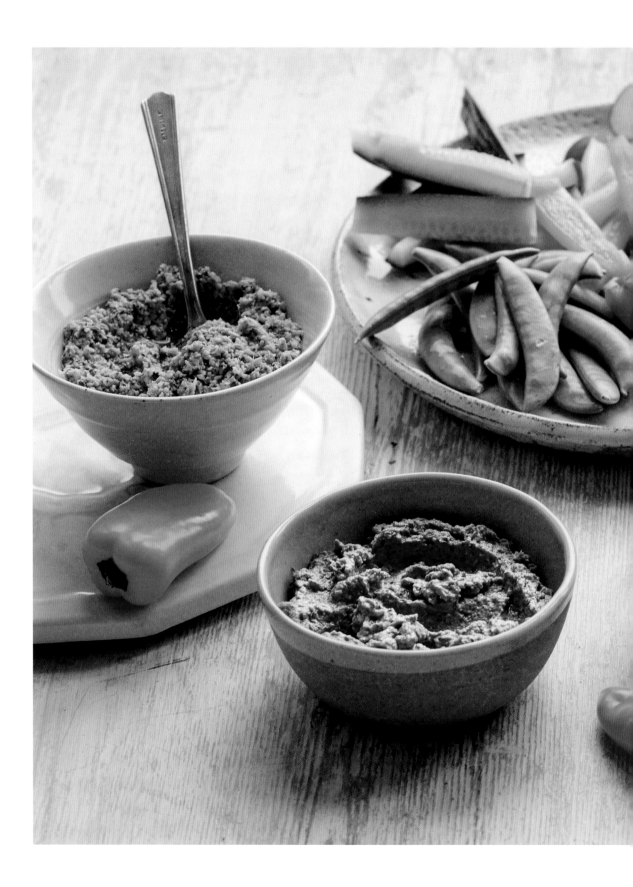

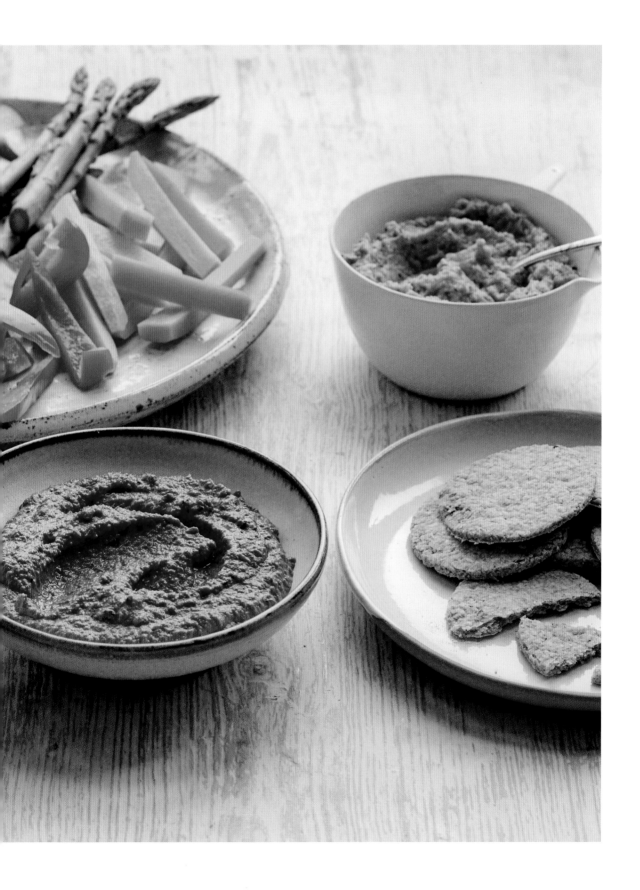

FIG ROLL OAT BARS

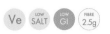

MAKES 16

When I came up with this recipe, I wanted to make a quick no-bake flapjack, but once I tasted it, it reminded me of the fig rolls I used to love with a cup of tea when growing up. I would get through half a packet easily if I was left to my own devices! The reason it's so easy to hoover up a pack of shop-bought biscuits is because they're relatively low in fibre, so they don't fill you up. They're also the 'perfect' combination of fat and sugar, so you keep going back for more. Well, I hope you will find this recipe just as moreish, but much more satisfying

Figs and oats are both high in fibre, so if you're feeling a little bloated (and maybe a little 'backed up'), this quick snack might just do the trick. People tend either to love figs or hate them, so if you're in the latter camp, you can use dates instead. Similarly, dried apricots are a good substitute for the raisins.

250g dried figs
100g raisins
100g flaked almonds
2 tbsp pumpkin seeds
150g oats
1 tsp ground cinnamon
1 tsp ground nutmeg

Line an 18cm square baking tin with baking parchment.

Place all the ingredients in a blender or food processor and blitz until they form a sticky dough.

Press the mixture firmly and evenly into the prepared tin. I find a good way of doing this is to cover it with clingfilm and press down with the back of a wooden spoon.

Cover and place in the fridge for 1 hour, or in the freezer for 30 minutes. When set, cut into 16 squares and store in an airtight container for up to 5 days.

VARIATION: *To make these bars a little more special, drizzle melted dark chocolate on top and sprinkle with flaked almonds.*

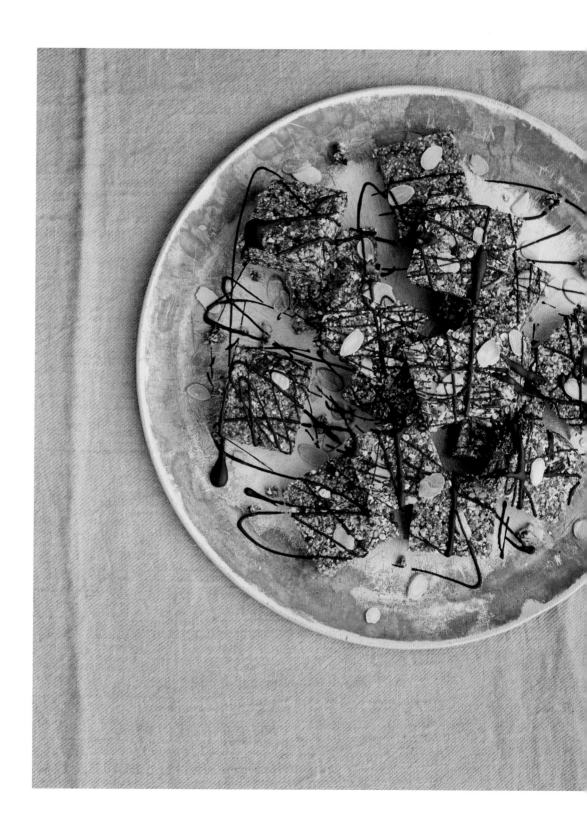

IS FIVE-A-DAY ENOUGH?

In the UK, and in many countries across the world, it is recommended that we eat a minimum of 400g, or five portions, of fruit and vegetables every day. These recommendations are based on advice from the World Health Organization, as evidence shows that high fruit and vegetable consumption can reduce the risk of certain cancers and cardiovascular disease (heart disease and stroke).

A study in 2017 investigated the optimal intake of fruit and vegetables that we need each day to get the best protection against disease and early death. The researchers pooled together ninety-five large studies, which included over two million people, to look at fruit and vegetable intake and the risk of various diseases.

They found that 10 portions (800g) of fruit and vegetables is associated with:

- *24% reduced risk of coronary heart disease*
- *33% reduced risk of stroke*
- *28% reduced risk of cardiovascular disease*
- *13% reduced risk of total cancer*
- *31% reduced risk of premature disease*

This risk was calculated in comparison to not eating any fruit and vegetables.

SO SHOULD YOU BE AIMING FOR TEN A DAY?

Essentially, this research backs up what most of us already know – the more fruit and vegetables in your diet, the better. However, in the UK only 27% of adults and 8% of children manage to meet even the current five-a-day target, so increasing that target to ten portions is quite an ambitious ask.

Furthermore, although the research suggests that increasing our fruit and veg intake beyond five portions a day can further reduce our risk of disease and early death, there are a number of things that may have influenced the results. Those who eat more fruit and vegetables are likely to be more health-conscious individuals, and therefore may be more physically active and avoid health-risk behaviours such as smoking and drinking alcohol. We call this 'healthy-user bias'. In addition, as with many studies looking at dietary habits, the researchers relied on self-reporting of food intake by the participants in the study, which is not always accurate or reliable.

Bottom line? I would advise aiming for at least 5–7 portions a day, and any more is a bonus. It might sound overwhelming, particularly if you're struggling to hit five portions already, but I've a few tips and tricks to help you boost your intake effortlessly.

WHAT COUNTS AS FIVE-A-DAY?

One portion is 80g of fresh, tinned or frozen fruit and vegetables, or 30g of dried fruit. This might look as follows:

- 1 medium banana
- ½ avocado
- 1 slice of a large fruit, such as a melon
- 2 satsumas
- 2 handfuls of blueberries
- 1 heaped tablespoon dried fruit
- 1 bowl of salad leaves
- 3 heaped tablespoons carrots
- ½ a large courgette

- 3 heaped tablespoons beans and pulses (Note that beans and pulses count as a maximum of one portion a day, however much you eat, because while they contain fibre, they don't give the same mixture of vitamins, minerals and other nutrients as fruit and vegetables.)

- 150ml unsweetened 100% fruit or vegetable juice or smoothie (No matter how much you drink, e.g. more than 150ml, or how many varieties of fruit juice, it will still count as only one of your portions per day because the juicing process removes most of the fibre. Also, fruit juices are a concentrated source of sugar.)

HOW TO MEET YOUR FIVE-A-DAY (AND MORE)

If you try to eat one or two portions with each meal, and make fruit or vegetables the first choice for a snack, it will be easy to eat at least five a day.

Sample day

BREAKFAST: 2 poached eggs, 1 grilled tomato, 4 tablespoons wilted spinach, 1 slice of rye bread

SNACK: 1 banana

LUNCH: A chopped salad of feta cheese (or vegan/vegetarian alternative), cherry tomatoes, broccoli, black olives and spinach

SNACK: Carrot and celery sticks with hummus

DINNER: Oven-baked salmon, roasted bell peppers and courgette, and homemade sweet potato wedges

DESSERT: 2 handfuls of blueberries and a pot of natural yogurt (or vegan/vegetarian alternative) with honey or maple syrup

Tips and tricks

- Sneak veggies into your diet – grated carrot or courgette in porridge, and blended fruit and vegetables in smoothies and juices.

- Snack on fruit and vegetables instead of biscuits and cakes.

- Use salads as the perfect opportunity to get a wide variety of vegetables in one meal.

- Omelettes and stir-fries are awesome vehicles for veggies, particularly leftover veg.

- Sweet potatoes count as one of your five-a-day (see page 17, where I show you ten different ways you can cook with them).

- Swap half your meat dish for veggies – chillis, stews, casseroles and curries are great opportunities to include more vegetables.

- Slurp on soup – add whatever you like to the mix: carrots, onions, sweet potatoes, parsnips and more. Either leave the soup chunky so it's more like a stew, or blitz until smooth (especially if you have fussy eaters to feed).

- Make your own pasta sauces with tinned tomatoes – this not only counts as one of your five-a-day, but also reduces the salt and sugar content that you would find in a ready-made sauce.

TRAIL MIX BARS

MAKES 18–20

This is the perfect snack to have in your bag on a busy day. Packed full of healthy fats and protein from the nuts and seeds, and energy from the oats and dried fruit, you'll be ticking things off your list like there's no tomorrow.

160g mixed seeds, e.g. pumpkin, sunflower, flax and chia

60g raw almonds, chopped

60g raw cashew nuts, chopped

60g raw pistachio nuts, chopped

60g oats

80g maple syrup

40g dried apricots, chopped

40g sultanas

65g cashew butter

50g coconut oil, melted

¼ tsp salt

Preheat the oven to 200°C/400°F/gas mark 6. Line an 18 x 24cm tin with baking parchment.

Spread the seeds, nuts and oats out in a baking tray and place in the oven for 6–8 minutes, until a shade darker and aromatic. Set aside to cool.

Once cool, transfer to a large mixing bowl, add the rest of the ingredients and stir until evenly mixed.

Put the mixture into the prepared tin and flatten it with the back of a spoon until smooth and compact.

Cover and place in the fridge for 1–2 hours, or in the freezer for 20 minutes, When set, cut into 18–20 bars or squares, then store in an airtight container in the fridge for up to 2 weeks.

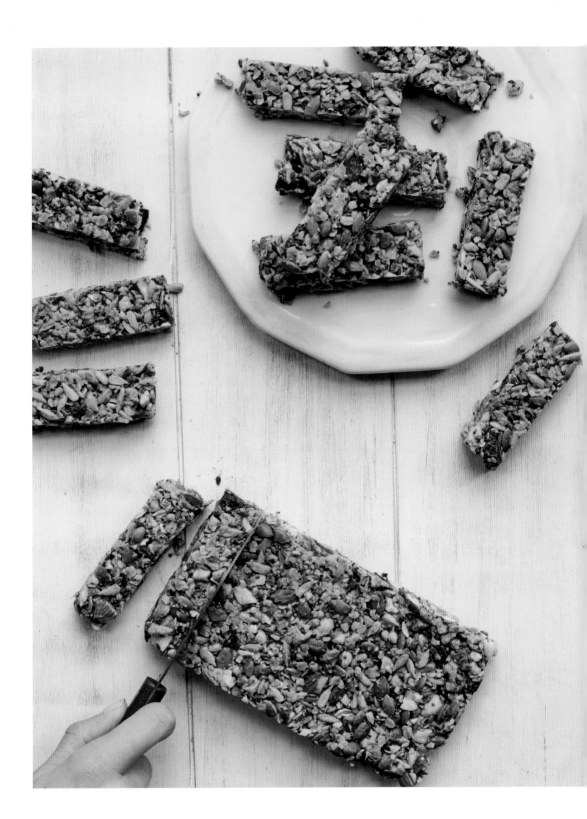

HAZELNUTTER BALLS

MAKES 8–10

I'm not going to claim that these are better than Ferrero Rocher chocolates, but they taste and smell very similar. The big difference is that you need only four ingredients to make these little guys, and they are pretty low in sugar, with about one and a half dates per ball. If you want to be super-fancy, roll the finished balls in melted chocolate and dip into crushed toasted hazelnuts for the full effect – ooh la la!

80g blanched hazelnuts

12 soft or medjool dates
(if they feel hard, soak in
hot water for 20 minutes
before use)

1 tbsp peanut butter

1 tbsp cocoa powder

Preheat the oven to 180°C/350°F/gas mark 4.

Place the hazelnuts in a baking tray and roast for 8–10 minutes, until golden.

Transfer the nuts to a blender or food processor, add all the remaining ingredients and blitz until the mixture starts to form a crumb. Add a dash of water if it feels too dry, or extra cocoa powder if it is too wet.

Scoop out spoonfuls of the mixture, squeeze to firm up, then roll into balls.

Put the balls on a tray and place in the fridge for 1 hour, or the freezer for 30 minutes before eating. They will keep in an airtight container in the fridge for about a week.

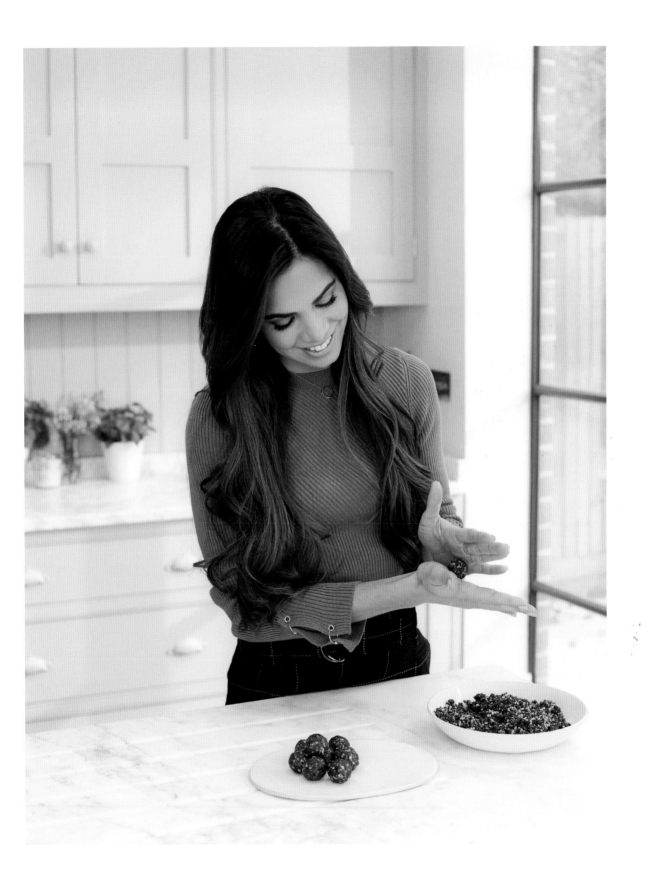

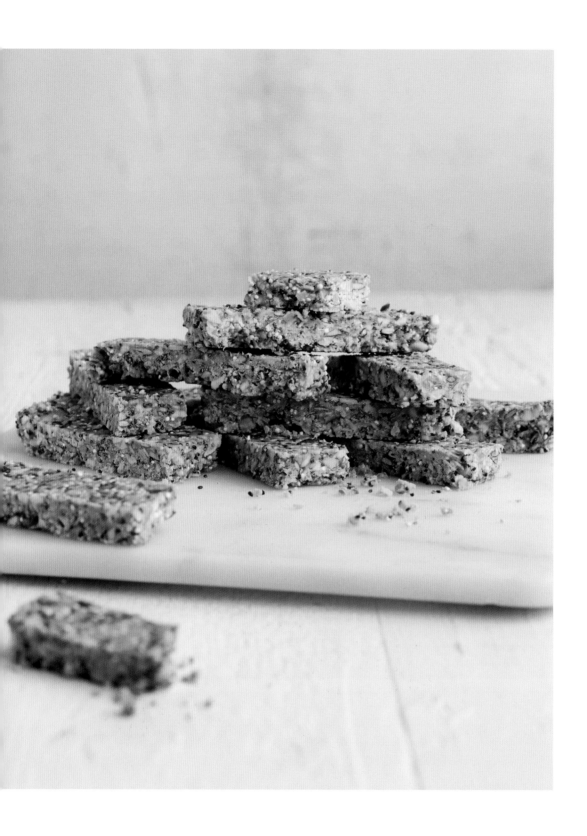

HOMEMADE PROTEIN BARS

MAKES 18–20

You'll find no protein powder in these lovely bars. Instead, I use high-protein plant sources such as quinoa, nuts and seeds. I've calculated over 6g of protein per bar – a perfect mid-afternoon snack before the gym.

50g raw quinoa
50g chia seeds
50g pumpkin seeds
80g cashew nuts
100g oats
150g crunchy peanut butter
50g honey or maple syrup
50ml coconut oil, melted
1 tsp vanilla extract
¼ tsp salt

Preheat the oven to 200°C/400°F/gas mark 6. Line an 18 x 24cm tin with baking parchment.

Spread the quinoa, seeds, nuts and oats out in a baking tray and place in the oven for 6–8 minutes, until a shade darker and aromatic. Set aside to cool for a few minutes, then place in a blender or food processor and pulse a few times until coarsely ground.

Transfer the seed and nut mixture to a large bowl, add the remaining ingredients and mix well.

Put the mixture into the prepared tin and flatten out with the back of a spoon until smooth and compact.

Cover and place in the fridge for 1–2 hours, or in the freezer for 20 minutes. When set, cut into 18–20 bars or squares, then store in an airtight container in the fridge for up to 2 weeks.

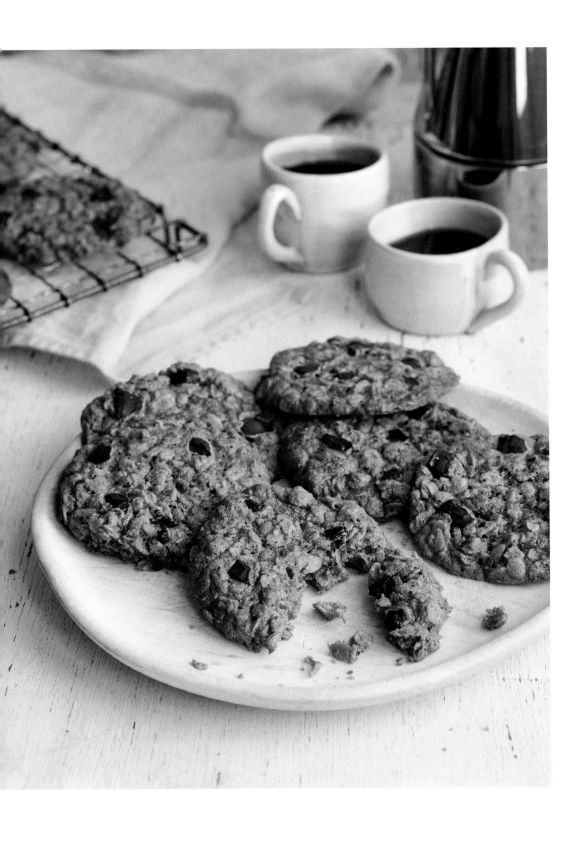

CHOCOLATE CHIP OATMEAL COOKIES

MAKES 12–14

Oatmeal cookies are my favourite type of biscuit, so much so that I've included a recipe for them in each of my books to date. This one is slightly different in terms of taste and texture, so I'll let you decide which one you prefer. Feel free to swap the chocolate for raisins or chopped nuts.

160g oats

65g white spelt flour

1 tsp ground cinnamon

½ tsp baking powder

¼ tsp salt

110g unsalted butter
  or coconut oil, at
  room temperature

110g brown sugar or
  coconut palm sugar

1 free-range egg

1½ tsp vanilla extract

75g dark chocolate chips or
  chopped dark chocolate

Preheat the oven to 180°C/350°F/gas mark 4 and line 2 baking trays with baking parchment.

Spread the oats out in a baking tray and toast in the oven for 15 minutes, until golden. Set aside to cool.

Meanwhile, put the flour, cinnamon, baking powder and salt into a bowl and mix together.

Put the butter into a separate bowl with the sugar, egg and vanilla and whisk at a high speed until light and fluffy. Reduce the speed to low, add the dry ingredients from the other bowl and whisk until just combined. Stir in the roasted oats and chocolate chips until evenly distributed.

Place heaped tablespoons of the mixture on the prepared trays, spacing them 2–3cm apart. Bake for 10–12 minutes, until golden and textured on top. If you prefer crispy rather than chewy biscuits, leave them in the oven for another 2 minutes.

Set aside to cool for 10 minutes, then carefully transfer to a wire rack to cool completely.

Serve immediately or store in an airtight container for up to 3 days.

CHOCOLATE-COATED RICE CAKES

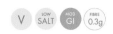

MAKES 6

I always used to buy chocolate rice cakes to snack on, until one day it dawned on me . . . why not make my own? So I did and I've never looked back. They're really fun to make and decorate, so an easy way to get kids involved in cooking.

6 squares (60g) dark
   chocolate (80–90%
   cocoa solids)

6 unsalted rice or
   corn cakes

FOR THE TOPPINGS

Flaked almonds

Chopped nuts

Coconut

Dried fruit

Seeds

Mulberries

Line a large plate or baking sheet with baking parchment.

Choose a bowl with a base that a rice cake can fit into. Melt the chocolate in the bowl over a saucepan of simmering water, or in the microwave for 20–30 seconds on full power.

Once the chocolate has melted, remove from the heat and dip a rice cake into the bowl. Transfer to the prepared plate or sheet and sprinkle with your chosen toppings. Repeat this step with each rice cake.

Place the rice cakes in the fridge for 10–15 minutes so that the chocolate hardens.

Eat immediately or store in an airtight container for 3–4 days.

TIP: *For the highest amount of polyphenols (see page 81), choose dark chocolate over milk or white chocolate. The percentage of chocolate on the label is an indicator of how much sugar is in it. So a 70% bar of dark chocolate is 70% cocoa solids and 30% sugar. Compare this to white chocolate, which contains zero cocoa solids and therefore zero polyphenols. The high fat and sugar content of white chocolate also makes it super easy to over-consume!*

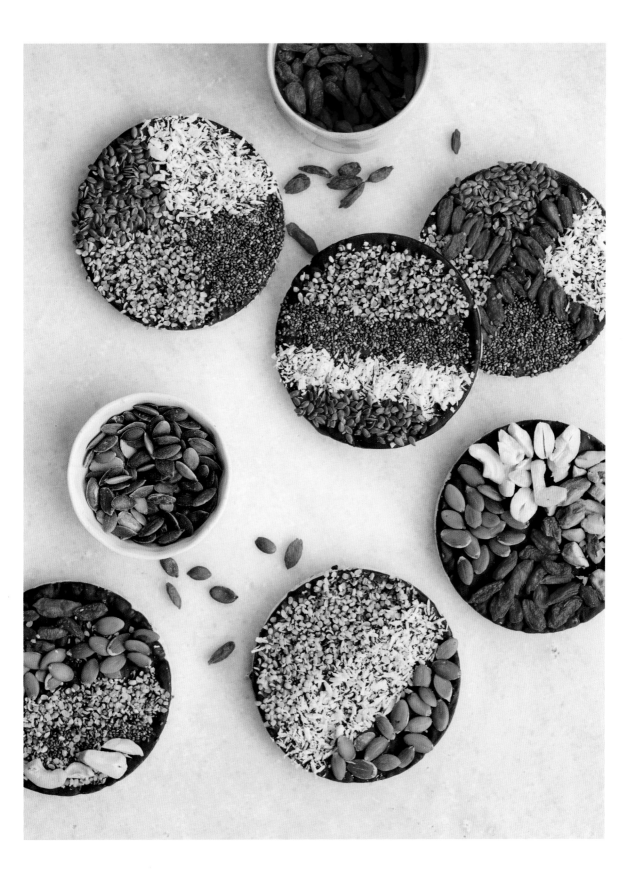

NO-RECIPE RECIPES

I think of these as my emergency snacks because I can knock them up quickly and take them to work with me, or nibble on them when I'm working from home. They are so simple that they're hardly recipes at all, hence the name.

TRAIL MIX

Mix together a small handful of chopped nuts, dried fruit and a chopped square of dark chocolate.

PEANUT BUTTER + JELLY-STUFFED DATES

Slice 12 medjool dates in half lengthways. Spoon ½ teaspoon peanut butter and ½ teaspoon Blueberry Chia Jam (see page 241) into each one.

APPLE RINGS + NUT BUTTER

Core the apple, then slice it widthways into rings about 1cm thick. Spread each slice with nut butter and sprinkle with seeds.

THREE-INGREDIENT COOKIES

Preheat the oven to 180°C/350°F/gas mark 4. Line a baking sheet with baking parchment. Place 100g oats in a bowl, then mix in 2 mashed ripe bananas. Stir in a handful of nuts or raisins or chocolate chips. Dot about 10 tablespoons of the mixture on the prepared sheet, spacing them about 2–3cm apart. Bake for 12–15 minutes, until golden.

SWEET + SPICY CHICKPEA CROUTONS

Preheat the oven to 180°C/350°F/gas mark 4. Drain and rinse a 400g tin of chickpeas. Place in a bowl, add 1 tablespoon oil, 1 teaspoon smoked paprika and ground cinnamon, ¼ teaspoon salt and toss well. Transfer to a baking tray and roast for 20–30 minutes, until golden.

FRUIT + NUT CHOCOLATE BARK

Melt 100g dark chocolate in a bowl set over a saucepan of simmering water, or in the microwave for 20–30 seconds on full power. Pour into a shallow baking tin lined with baking parchment. Sprinkle with chopped nuts and dried fruit, then place in the fridge to set. Break into pieces and eat.

BERRY FRO-YO

Place 2 handfuls of frozen berries in a blender or food processor, add a small tub of natural or coconut yogurt, a tablespoon of maple syrup or honey and blitz for 20–30 seconds.

CHICKPEA COOKIE DOUGH

Drain and rinse a 400g tin of chickpeas. Place in a blender or food processor and add 120g peanut butter, 3 tablespoons maple syrup and 1 teaspoon vanilla extract. Blitz until smooth, then stir in a hanfdul of chocolate chips. Transfer the mixture to a bowl. Keep in the fridge and eat on its own or with oatcakes, ice cream or even on porridge.

CRUDITÉS + DIP

Cut up sticks of carrot, celery and cucumber and eat them with a homemade dip (see pages 130–131).

SWEET POTATO TOAST

Preheat the oven to 200°C/400°F/gas mark 6. Peel a sweet potato, then cut lengthways into slices 1cm thick. Place in a roasting tin and roast for 20 minutes. Spread with your favourite toppings, perhaps peanut butter and chia jam, fig and goat's cheese, or smashed avocado and egg.

POWER DOWN

People often ask me, 'How do you do it all? How can you possibly fit everything you do as a doctor, an author, a social media personality and a businesswoman into a day?' It's true – I have a lot going on in my life. We all do. Most people, when asked, will say they have a busy life, regardless of what job(s) they do, how many kids or parents they look after, or the extent of their social activities. The prospect of fitting in time for ourselves to unwind can send many of us into a frenzy of stress and panic.

However, we can all find a little calm, even in the craziest of schedules, and I'm going to show you how. I often find that cooking offers me a moment of peace even in the busiest days. I hope that these recipes encourage you to get lost in the process and use cooking as almost a form of mindfulness and relaxation. You can also turn to pages 192 and 238 for the lowdown on calming your mind and resting your body.

TOO BUSY TO REST

We all need to create more space in our lives. This might seem impossible for the working mum of three, or the university student juggling a full-time degree and a part-time job. You might be thinking that I couldn't possibly understand how busy you are.

I may not have kids yet, and I've finished my university education, but I do know what it feels like to be completely overwhelmed with how busy I am. I know what it is to feel that there are not enough hours in the day, to feel like I'm not on top of my to-do list, to feel like any spare minute must be filled with something 'productive', such as checking emails or cramming in work, to feel so incredibly busy that simple things, such as cooking dinner or washing my hair, seem less of a priority than meeting a work deadline.

I know. I know. I know.

Well, we can't quit our jobs or sell the kids, but we can learn to cut down on the things that suck out our energy and don't serve us, including the stress we put on ourselves.

We can learn to say no, and not feel guilty for it. We can schedule some daily calm into our day through breathing techniques and meditation. We can switch off our apps, smart phones, smart watches and other devices, and choose when we look at them – not allow them to demand our attention through constant push notifications and vibrations. We can improve our sleep regime and go to bed an hour earlier, achieving a more restful sleep and, overall, a less stressed state of mind.

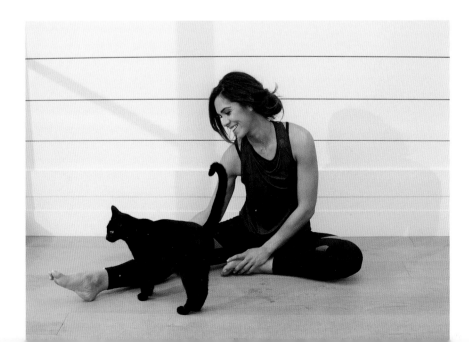

BRUNCHES

To my mind, weekends are made for baking and brunches (and a little laundry). There is such a wonderful brunch scene these days that I love nothing more than spending my Sunday mornings catching up with friends over coffee and a delicious late breakfast/early lunch.

Brunch at home, though, means no waiting in line, as many cups of coffee as your heart desires, and, best of all, eating in your pyjamas. This chapter has something for everyone, whether your preference is for sweet or savoury, and the recipes, of course, are super-easy . . . easy like Sunday morning.

SMOKED SALMON-WRAPPED ASPARAGUS WITH POACHED EGGS + TOMATOES

SERVES 2

This breakfast sounds and looks far more fancy and complicated than it is. It's also very low in sugar, so is suitable for diabetics who are looking for a satisfying breakfast that won't play havoc with their blood sugar.

1 tbsp olive oil

8 asparagus spears

10 cherry tomatoes, halved

1 tbsp cream cheese

2 tsp horseradish sauce

8 slices of smoked salmon

2 large handfuls of
  rocket leaves

A dash of white wine
  vinegar

2 free-range eggs

Salt and black pepper

Place the oil in a frying pan over a medium heat. When hot, add the asparagus spears and fry for about 4–5 minutes, until tender and lightly crisp. Add the tomatoes for the final minute and toss in the pan to warm through. Season with salt and pepper.

Put the cream cheese and horseradish in a bowl and mix well. Spread this mixture on one side of the salmon slices. Wrap each slice around an asparagus spear, cheese side inwards.

Divide the rocket leaves between two plates and top with the asparagus spears and tomatoes.

Bring a pan of water to the boil. Add a dash of white wine vinegar, then lower the heat to a simmer. Stir once to create a 'whirlpool'. Crack an egg into a cup or ramekin and slide it into the water – the whirlpool will help to form it into a neat shape. Cook for 3–4 minutes if you want a soft yolk. Lift out with a slotted spoon and drain on kitchen paper. Repeat with the other egg.

To serve, place the egg on top of the asparagus. Sprinkle with salt and pepper and serve straight away.

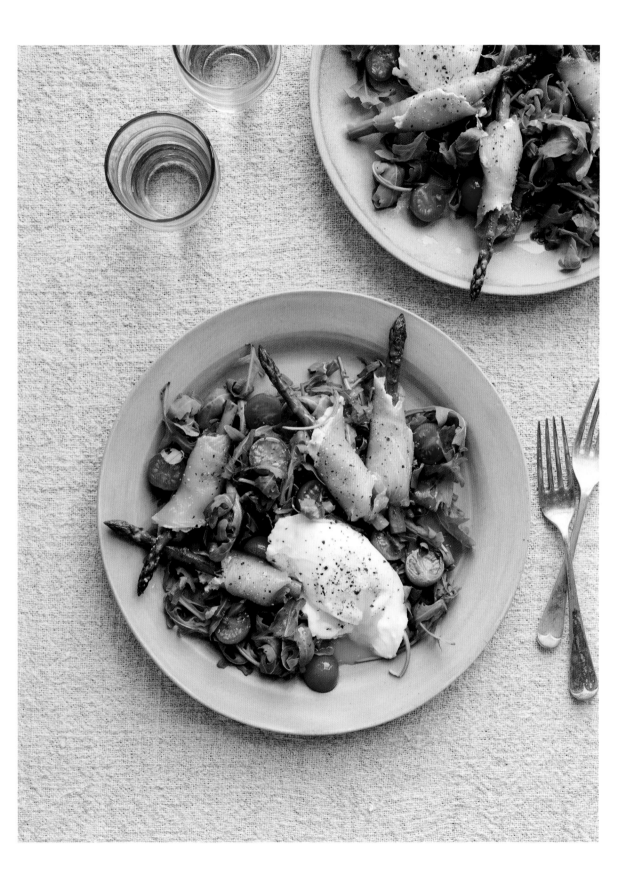

POACHED EGGS + SWEET
POTATO FRITTERS

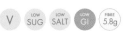

SERVES 4

Personally, I'm tired of being offered smashed avocado on toast everywhere I go for brunch these days. It's time to think outside the breakfast box and start making our own brunch feasts at home. As far as I'm concerned, nothing says brunch quite like poached eggs and sweet potato fritters.

500g sweet potato, peeled and coarsely grated

½ onion, very finely chopped

3 garlic cloves, crushed

50g spelt flour

6 free-range eggs, 2 of them beaten together

Zest of 1 lemon

15g Parmesan cheese, finely grated (optional)

Large handful of flat-leaf parsley leaves, finely chopped

1 tsp ground coriander

1 tbsp sunflower oil, to fry

Extra-virgin olive oil, to drizzle

Salt and black pepper

Place the sweet potato in a large bowl with the onion, garlic, flour, beaten eggs, lemon zest, Parmesan (if using), most of the parsley, the ground coriander and 1 teaspoon salt. Mix well.

Put the oil in a frying pan over a medium heat. When hot, add 3 or 4 heaped tablespoons of the sweet potato mix, spacing them out and flattening them gently into rough circles. Fry for 5–6 minutes on each side until crisp and golden. Remove and keep warm while you make the rest.

Poach the eggs for 3–4 minutes (see page 154). Using a slotted spoon, lift out the eggs and drain them on kitchen paper.

To serve, plate up the fritters with a poached egg on top and sprinkle with the remaining parsley. Drizzle over a little olive oil and season with salt and pepper. Serve immediately.

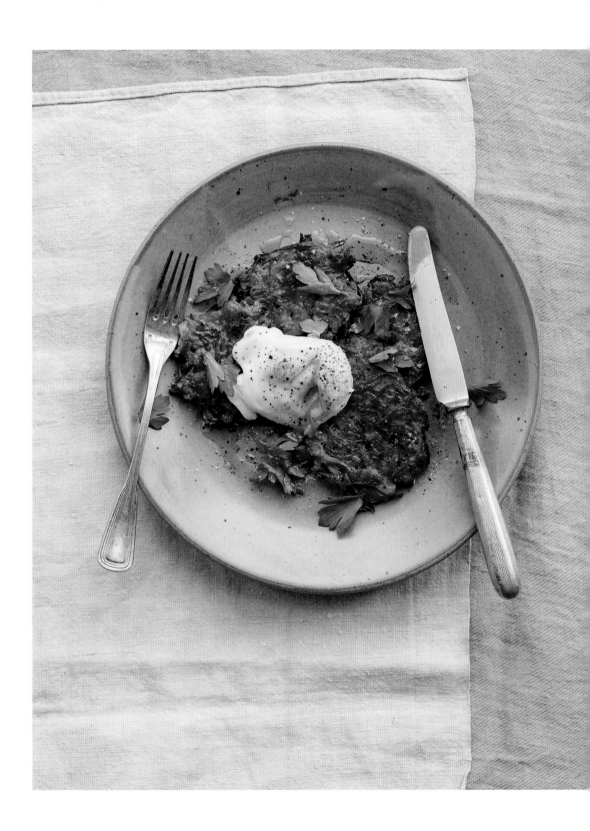

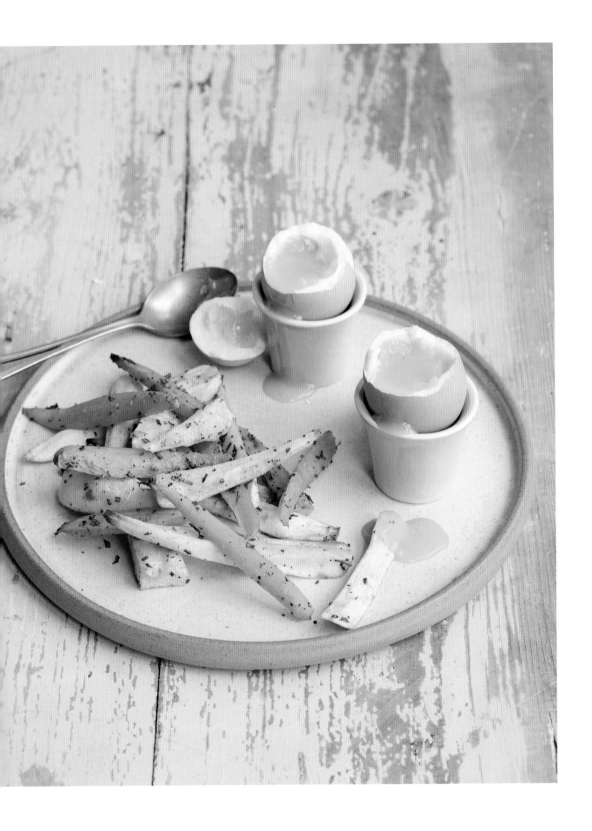

DIPPY EGGS + ROOT
VEGETABLE SOLDIERS

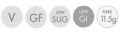

SERVES 2

This is a slightly more sophisticated twist on the childhood classic with toast soldiers. My mum used to make me boiled eggs and toast on the days I had to stay home from school because I was ill. She would serve it up with gorgeous buttery toast and a big mug of tea. 'Feed a cold, starve a fever,' she used to say, but I think she used to feed us up regardless of our state of health. She was the first person to plant the seed in my head that food was indeed a form of medicine.

2 carrots, ideally different colours (see tip below), peeled and sliced lengthways

2 parsnips, peeled and sliced lengthways

1 tbsp olive oil

1 tbsp chopped fresh rosemary

¼ tsp salt

¼ tsp black pepper

4 free-range eggs, at room temperature

Preheat the oven to 200°C/400°F/gas mark 6. Line a baking sheet with baking parchment.

Place the vegetables in a large bowl. Add the oil, rosemary, salt and pepper and toss to coat.

Arrange the vegetables on the prepared baking sheet and roast for 30–35 minutes, turning halfway through.

To boil the eggs, gently lower them into a pan of boiling water one at a time. Cook for 6 minutes if you like a runny yolk (that's my preference for this recipe), 7–8 minutes for semi-firm, and 10 minutes for hard-boiled.

Lift out the eggs using a slotted spoon and place them in egg cups. Crack the top off the eggs and serve with the vegetable soldiers.

TIP: *If you can get your hands on different-coloured carrots, this breakfast will be even more special in terms of appearance and nutritional profile.*

THE FOOD MEDIC FRY-UP

SERVES 1

There is nothing I love more at the weekend than making a really awesome brunch. A traditional fry-up is often devoid of vegetables – well, you might get a spoonful of beans or a grilled tomato – and tends to be focused on eggs, sausages and bacon served up with toast or hash browns. Although there is absolutely nothing wrong with that selection, I think a fry-up can be taken up a notch in terms of taste and nutritional value with the addition of a few veg. The quantities in this recipe can easily be multiplied, depending on how many mouths you have to feed.

1½ tbsp oil or butter

¼ red onion, thinly sliced

5 tenderstem broccoli tips

Handful of button mushrooms, halved

Handful of cherry tomatoes, halved

1 slice of rye or sourdough bread

1 or 2 free-range eggs (depending on appetite)

30g feta cheese (optional)

¼ tsp chilli flakes

Salt and black pepper

Place a tablespoon of the oil in a large frying pan over a medium heat. When hot, fry the onion for 1–2 minutes, until soft.

Add the broccoli tips and mushrooms and cook for 5 minutes, until golden.

Add the tomatoes and cook for a further 2 minutes. Sprinkle with salt and pepper and transfer to a serving plate.

Toast the bread. Meanwhile, put the frying pan back on a medium heat and add ½ tablespoon oil. As soon as it is hot, carefully break in the egg, then lower the heat and fry until the white is translucent and the yolk is cooked to your liking. I like mine runny, so I usually cook it for 1–2 minutes. Remove the pan from the heat and transfer the egg to a plate.

Place the vegetable mixture beside it, then crumble the feta on top (if using). Sprinkle the chilli flakes over the egg and eat with your buttered toast.

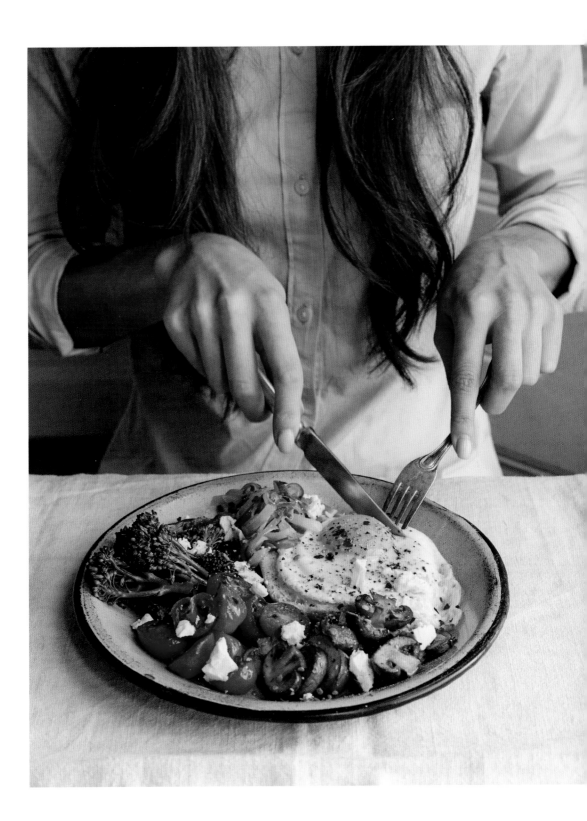

SHAKSHUKA EGGS
+ CRUMBLED FETA

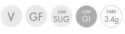

SERVES 3

It blows most people's minds that a couple of eggs and a tin of tomatoes can be transformed into this bubbling pan of gooey goodness. If serving just two people, use fewer eggs and mop up the extra sauce with crusty bread.

1 tbsp olive oil

1 small onion, diced

2 garlic cloves, grated

1 green or red pepper, deseeded and chopped

Handful of cherry tomatoes (about 10) or 2 large ripe tomatoes

1 x 400g tin of chopped tomatoes

2 tbsp tomato purée

1 tsp ground cumin

1 tsp smoked paprika

¼ tsp chilli flakes

¼ tsp salt

Pinch of sugar (optional)

Handful of spinach

6 free-range eggs

60g feta cheese

1 tbsp freshly chopped parsley (optional)

Salt and black pepper

Place the oil in a large frying pan over a medium heat. When hot, fry the onion for a few minutes until it begins to soften. Add the garlic and continue to fry until soft and translucent. Add the bell pepper and fry for 3–5 minutes, until softened.

Stir in the tomatoes and tomato purée, then add the spices, salt and sugar (if using). Simmer the mixture over a medium heat for about 5 minutes, until it starts to reduce. Toss in the spinach and stir together.

Make little wells in the sauce, making sure to space them evenly, and crack an egg into each one. Cook for 5–10 minutes, depending on how soft you like your yolks. To speed up the process you can pop the pan under a hot grill, provided the pan is flameproof.

Crumble the feta on top, season to taste and sprinkle with the parsley (if using). Serve with crusty sourdough bread or a simple side salad.

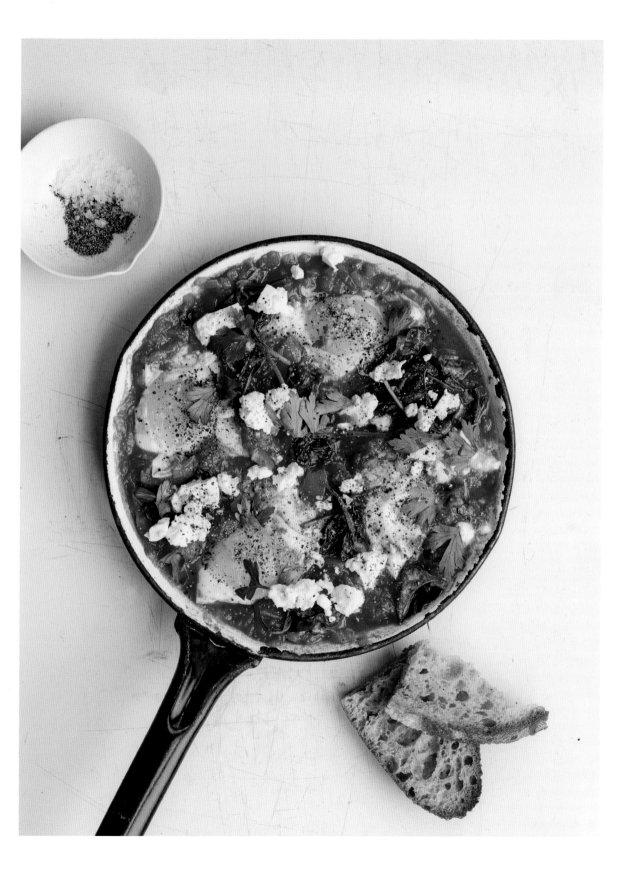

VEGETARIAN + VEGAN DIETS

Switching towards a more plant-focused diet, i.e. becoming a vegetarian or vegan, is very much on trend at the moment. The reason for adopting a plant-based diet could be one of many: ethical or environmental issues, cultural or religious beliefs, or perceived health benefits. Personally, I am not vegan or vegetarian. Eating meat is part of my heritage and I don't have any moral dilemmas about eating well-sourced meat and fish. As a doctor, I wouldn't advise patients to change their diet to vegan or vegetarian in order to improve their health, but I would advise everyone to include more plant foods in their diet.

To clarify terms, when I refer to 'plant-based', I'm using this as an umbrella term for both vegetarian and vegan. Although vegetarians eat primarily plant foods, they also consume eggs and dairy produce. A vegan, though, eliminates all animal products – meat, fish, dairy and eggs – and focuses entirely on plant foods. Most other people, myself included, are omnivores, which means we consume a variety of animal foods (meat, fish and dairy), but also include plant foods (fruit, vegetables, grains and legumes).

The debate as to whether a plant-based diet is healthier than an omnivorous diet is extremely complex and beyond the scope of this book. Dietary choices are very personal to each individual. However, I believe if the two camps stopped wasting time throwing rocks at one another and opened up the conversation, we would discover that there is a lot to learn from both sides.

PROS AND CONS

A leading concern regarding a plant-based diet, particularly a vegan diet, is that there is a higher risk of nutrient deficiencies. Nutrients that are a bit trickier to obtain from vegetarian and vegan diets include iron and zinc, calcium, vitamins B12 and D, and omega 3 fatty acids. Adequate intake of complete protein sources (i.e. proteins that contain all nine essential amino acids) is also slightly more difficult for a plant-based eater, but less problematic for vegetarians compared to vegans, as eggs and dairy are complete sources of protein.

On the other hand, vegetarian and vegan diets tend to be richer than omnivorous diets in other nutrients, such as fibre, folic acid, vitamins C and E, potassium and magnesium, and contain less saturated fat. Increasing the amount of plant-based foods we eat automatically increases our intake of fibre, antioxidants and phytochemicals, and this in turn may reduce the risk of high blood pressure, raised blood cholesterol, stroke and heart disease.

Note that I say vegetarian and vegan diets 'tend to' be richer in other nutrients, as simply cutting out animal products does not mean you will have a nutrient-dense diet. It's still important to choose nutrient-dense foods, such as fruits and vegetables, legumes and wholegrains, rather than following the typical western fast-food diet minus the meat. Did you know Oreos are vegan? I rest my case.

GOING PLANT-BASED AND GETTING ENOUGH NUTRIENTS

Well-planned vegetarian and vegan diets can be incredibly nutritious and healthy because they tend to be lower in saturated fat, higher in fibre, and contain greater amounts of fruit and vegetables than omnivorous diets. However, there are a few nutrients that are slightly more difficult to obtain from plant-based, particularly vegan, diets, namely: complete protein sources, calcium, iron, omega 3 fatty acids vitamins B12 and D, and zinc. Let's look at each of these in turn.

PROTEIN

Generally, those on a plant-based diet are not at risk of protein deficiency, but it is more challenging to get complete protein sources through plant foods alone. Complete proteins are those that contain all the essential amino acids, i.e. those we can't make ourselves and must get from food. The main sources are animal foods (meat, fish and dairy), but plant-based sources include soya, quinoa, hemp and chia seeds. Most other plant proteins provide some, but not all, essential amino acids, with each plant providing a different combination. So as long as you're eating a mixture of different plant proteins, you'll be getting all the essential amino acids your body needs. Examples of how you might combine your plant-based proteins include eating hummus on rye bread, or serving Lentil + Kidney Bean Chilli (see page 115) with brown rice. In theory, therefore, a well-balanced, plant-based diet should provide all the essential amino acids.

PROTEIN SOURCES FOR VEGETARIANS AND VEGANS	
VEGETARIAN ONLY	VEGETARIAN + VEGAN
Eggs	Beans, lentils and chickpeas
Dairy (milk, cheese, yogurt)	Tofu and soya products
Whey protein	Vegan protein blends (hemp/pea/brown rice)
	Seeds, nuts and nut butters
	Wholegrains

Note: Most plant-based milks, such as almond, coconut and oat, are low in protein. Soy milk has the highest protein content.

IS RED MEAT BAD FOR YOU?

I know many of you reading this might be concerned about the reported link between red meat and cancer. Maybe you have read about it in the papers or online, or heard about it in a documentary. The problem with sensational headlines in the media is that they never tell the whole story, and they use over-the-top statements to grab people's attention.

In one online newspaper, within the space of one week, I came across two conflicting headlines: 'New cancer alert over eating just one steak a week' and 'Why red meat can be good for your health'. They were published one day apart. No wonder people are confused.

WELL, WHAT ARE THE FACTS, THEN, DOC?

At the moment the evidence is that eating red meat (beef, pork, lamb and goat) is a probable cause of colorectal cancer, and that eating processed red meat that has been smoked, cured or has added salt and preservatives (e.g. bacon, salami, corned beef, pepperoni, hot dogs and all types of ham) is a convincing cause of colorectal cancer. Note that processed meat does not include meat that has simply been pre-cooked or re-formed (like some burgers and sausages).

The World Cancer Research Fund advises us to reduce red meat consumption to 500g (cooked weight) per week, and to avoid processed meat entirely. The UK government has less stringent guidelines and simply advises a reduction of both red and processed meat consumption to 70g per day.

Wow! A lot to think about? Well, I wouldn't get bogged down on the numbers. Let's focus on quality over quantity.

I think we can all agree that it is wise for our own health, and for the health of the planet, to reduce our red meat consumption, and when we do choose to eat it, to choose good-quality, unprocessed meat from sustainably farmed sources.

CALCIUM

Provided they eat dairy and soya products, vegetarians should not have an issue getting adequate amounts of calcium through their diet. Vegans, though, may find it more difficult. Calcium absorption from plant foods is adversely affected by plant molecules called 'oxalates'. This means that while leafy greens such as spinach have a relatively high calcium content, the calcium is not efficiently absorbed during digestion. One study comparing calcium in plant foods to calcium in milk suggested that it would take sixteen servings of spinach to achieve the same amount of absorbable calcium found in a 240ml glass of milk. Other plant-based sources of calcium include fortified plant milks, nuts and seeds, tofu and tempeh, and leafy green vegetables, such as kale.

IRON

Iron is needed to make haemoglobin, which is a protein that transports oxygen around the body in the bloodstream. Low iron levels result in iron-deficiency anaemia, which can be caused by lack of iron in the diet, or blood loss during menstruation or from the gastrointestinal tract (which can be caused by ulcers or Crohn's disease).

SYMPTOMS OF ANAEMIA

- Constant fatigue
- Shortness of breath
- Pale skin or dark circles around the eyes
- Headache, dizziness or feeling light-headed
- Weakness
- Poor appetite

If you have some of these symptoms, it would be worth speaking to your GP, who can do a simple blood test to check your iron levels.

The best sources of iron come from animal products – red meat, fish and eggs. This is called haem iron and is easily absorbed by the body.

Although iron is abundant in plant foods, such as grains, legumes, nuts and seeds, the body finds it slightly more difficult to absorb from these sources. This non-haem iron must undergo a chemical change before it can be absorbed.

The absorption of iron is affected by other foods in the diet, including tea and coffee, and naturally occurring plant chemicals called 'phytates', which are found in nuts, legumes and grains. Phytates bind to and block the absorption of certain nutrients, particularly iron, zinc and calcium. In well-balanced diets, this is rarely a concern, but it may cause nutrient deficiencies in those who depend on plant-based foods for the majority of their calories and nutrients.

TIPS TO IMPROVE THE ABSORPTION OF NON-HAEM IRON

IRON-RICH FOODS FOR A PLANT-BASED DIET	
VEGETARIAN ONLY	VEGETARIAN + VEGAN
Egg yolks	Pulses (beans, lentils and chickpeas)
	Green leafy vegetables (spinach and kale)
	Fortified cereals and bread
	Nuts and seeds
	Dried fruit (apricots, dates and raisins)

- Vitamin C can increase the absorption of dietary iron, so try adding lemon or lime juice to your salad dressing, or bell peppers to your curries and stews.

- The phytic acid content of food can be reduced by using various preparation techniques, including soaking, sprouting and fermenting.

- Avoid drinking tea and coffee with meals, having them between instead.

Please note that phytates have lots of health benefits, so we shouldn't exclude them from our diet.

My take-away message to you? Unless the majority of your diet is made up of nuts, legumes and grains, you probably do not need to be concerned about having nutritional iron, zinc or calcium deficiencies. If you are concerned, you can always take the steps suggested above to reduce the amount of phytates in your diet, and aim to consume mineral-fortified foods, or consider taking mineral supplements if you have confirmed nutrient deficiencies diagnosed by your GP.

OMEGA 3 FATTY ACIDS

The omega 3 fatty acids include docosahexaenoic acid (DHA), eicosapentaenoic acid (EPA), and alpha linolenic acid (ALA). DHA and EPA are found in oily fish, such as salmon and mackerel, and it is advised that we eat two portions of fish per week, one oily, in order to get these essential nutrients. Obviously, vegetarian and vegan diets don't include fish, but ALA, which is found in plant foods such as flaxseeds, chia seeds and walnuts, can be used by the body to make EPA and DHA. However, the amount produced from ALA may not be enough, so it might be useful to include an omega 3 supplement.

VITAMIN B12

This vitamin is involved in the production of red blood cells and is also essential for the proper functioning and development of the brain and nerve cells. Just as with iron, a lack of vitamin B12 can lead to anaemia and shares the same symptoms (see opposite page), but deficiency can also lead to nerve damage, causing symptoms of pins and needles, a lack of sensation, and even mental health conditions such as depression and dementia.

Vitamin B12 occurs only in animal products, so vegetarians who eat eggs and dairy should not have to worry about being deficient. Vegans, however, cannot get B12 from plants, and are unlikely to get the total daily requirement from fortified foods, so they should take a supplement.

VITAMIN D

Our bodies make vitamin D from sunlight during the summer months (April–October), but outside these months the government recommends that everyone living in the UK take a supplement of 10 micrograms. Vegetarian sources rich in vitamin D include eggs, fortified margarines, breakfast cereals and soya milk.

ZINC

As an essential trace element, zinc plays a number of important roles in promoting good health: supporting the body's immune system, assisting in wound healing, hormone production and fertility, and the formation of important proteins. Symptoms of zinc deficiency range from hair loss and brittle nails to impaired wound healing and decreased fertility.

Just as with iron, phytates found in plant foods can reduce zinc absorption. Good plant-based sources of zinc include fermented soya (tempeh and miso); beans (soak and rinse dried beans before cooking them to increase zinc absorption); wholegrains, nuts, seeds and certain fortified breakfast cereals.

SPELT + BUCKWHEAT PANCAKES

**SERVES 2–3
(MAKES 6–8)**

I love to see a pile of pancakes in the centre of the table surrounded with various toppings so that people can dig in and help themselves. I first made this recipe when I had my sister come to stay, and she really fancied pancakes for Sunday brunch. It was one of those experiments that worked out an absolute treat, and now this recipe has become a staple of mine. The flavour is quite neutral, so the pancakes go well with both sweet and savoury options.

60g buckwheat flour

80g spelt flour

½ tsp baking powder

1 tsp ground cinnamon

1 free-range egg

200ml milk

1–2 tbsp honey or
   maple syrup

1 tsp vanilla extract

1 tbsp coconut oil or
   butter, melted, plus
   extra to grease

Salt

FOR THE TOPPINGS

Blueberry Chia Jam (see
   page 241), Greek yogurt
   and maple syrup

Chocolate, peanut butter
   and banana

Lemon juice, butter and
   maple syrup

Goat's cheese, toasted
   pecans and honey

Poached egg and
   smashed avocado

Sift the flours and baking powder into a large bowl. Add the cinnamon and a pinch of salt. Mix well with a whisk.

In a separate bowl, whisk together the egg, milk, honey, vanilla and melted coconut oil. Pour the mixture slowly into the bowl of dry ingredients, whisking to prevent lumps. If your mixture feels too dry, add more milk, although for these American-style pancakes, you don't want your batter very runny.

Place a large non-stick frying pan on a medium heat and grease with a little coconut oil. When hot, place 2–3 spoonfuls of the batter into the pan, spacing them apart. Cook for 1–2 minutes on each side, until golden. Set aside on a plate and keep warm while you cook the remaining pancakes.

Serve with your choice of toppings.

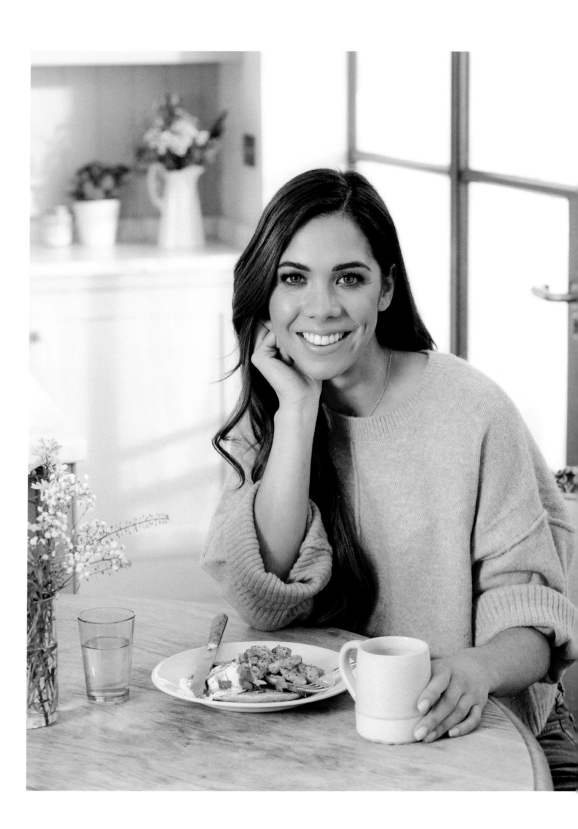

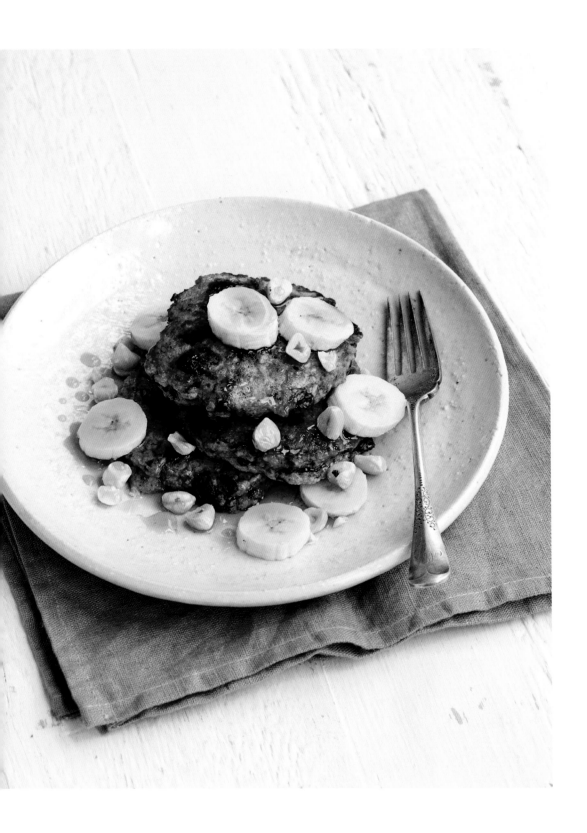

CHOCOLATE CHIP BANANA PANCAKES

**SERVES 2
(MAKES 6–8)**

This is one of the easiest, most foolproof pancake recipes you will ever make, and the ingredients are probably sitting in your cupboard already. Literally chuck all the ingredients in a blender, blitz them up and you're laughing. Perfect for both kids and adults alike.

1 ripe banana

2 free-range eggs

1 tbsp milk, plus extra
  if necessary

80g oats

1 tsp baking powder

50g dark chocolate
  chips or finely chopped
  chocolate

Coconut oil or butter,
  to grease

TO SERVE

1 banana, sliced

Maple syrup

2 tbsp toasted, chopped
  hazelnuts

Put the banana, eggs and milk in a blender and blitz for 10 seconds, until smooth.

Add the oats and baking powder and blend for another 10–20 seconds, until smooth and creamy. Add an extra tablespoon of milk if the mixture is too thick. Stir in the chocolate chips.

Place a large, non-stick frying pan on a medium heat and grease with the oil. When hot, place a ladleful of the batter into the pan. Cook for 1–2 minutes on each side, until golden. Repeat with the remaining batter.

Serve topped with the sliced banana, some maple syrup and chopped hazelnuts.

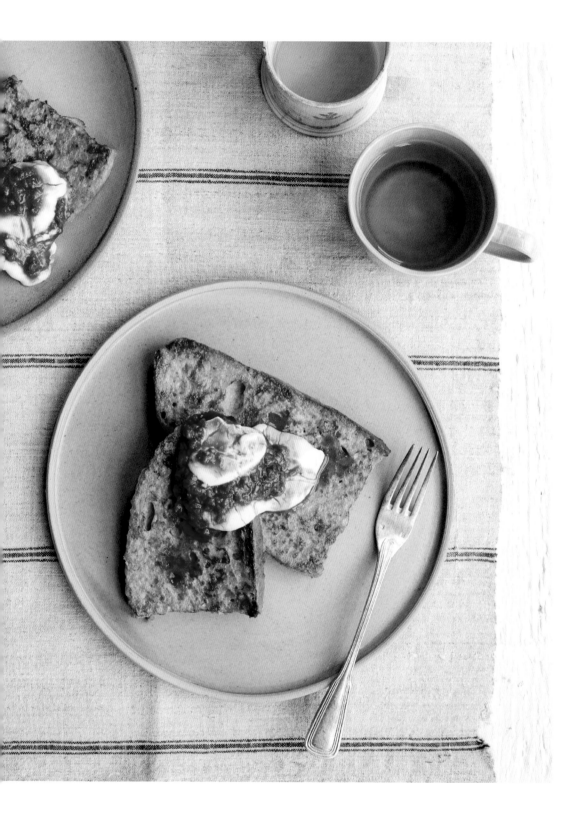

FRENCH TOAST WITH BERRY COMPOTE

SERVES 1

When growing up, our birthday breakfast was French toast, which my mum used to claim was the best way to get an egg into a child. This recipe is not far from the one we used at home, but I've omitted the sugar usually added to the egg mixture. To be honest, you don't miss it because the toppings tend to be sweet enough anyway.

1 large free-range egg
100ml milk
½ tsp vanilla extract
½ tsp ground cinnamon
Butter or coconut oil,
   to grease
2 slices of rye or
   sourdough bread

FOR THE COMPOTE
200g frozen berries
1 tbsp water
1 tbsp sugar

First make the compote. Tip the berries into a pan with the water and sugar. Cook gently over a medium heat until the berries are warm and mushy.

Crack the egg into a shallow dish, add the milk, vanilla and cinnamon, then whisk together until well combined.

Heat a non-stick frying pan over a medium heat and grease with a little butter or oil.

Dip the bread in the egg mixture, turning to coat both sides evenly. Place in the pan and fry for 2–3 minutes on each side, until lightly browned.

Serve with the compote spooned on top.

IRISH SWEET POTATO FARLS

MAKES 4

My grandmother lived in the very south of Ireland in Tipperary. She had a tiny two-bedroom cottage, where she raised my mum and her fifteen brothers and sisters. I used to love visiting her because she cooked such comforting food, including potato farls. These are basically a cross between a bread and a pancake, and they go well with eggs, jam or simply butter.

1 large baked sweet potato

250g white spelt flour, plus extra to dust

½ tsp salt

1 tsp bicarbonate of soda

135ml buttermilk

Cut open the baked sweet potato and scoop 150g of the flesh into a large bowl. (Save the remainder for use in soup or a salad.) Mash the flesh with a fork, then sift in the flour, salt and bicarbonate of soda and mix well. Pour in the buttermilk and mix again to form a thick and slightly sticky dough.

Dust your work surface with flour and tip the dough onto it. Knead briefly, just until the dough is smooth. Roll it into a ball, then flatten into a circle about 1.5cm thick. Using a floured knife, cut the circle into 4 equal triangles.

Place a dry, heavy-based frying pan over a medium heat. When hot, dust with a little flour to prevent sticking, then add the triangles of dough. Cook over a medium–low heat for 8–10 minutes on each side, until golden and cooked through. Take care not to have the heat too high or the farls will burn before they have cooked. Remove the pan from the heat and transfer to a wire rack to cool for 5 minutes.

Serve the farls cut in half horizontally and slathered with butter and jam.

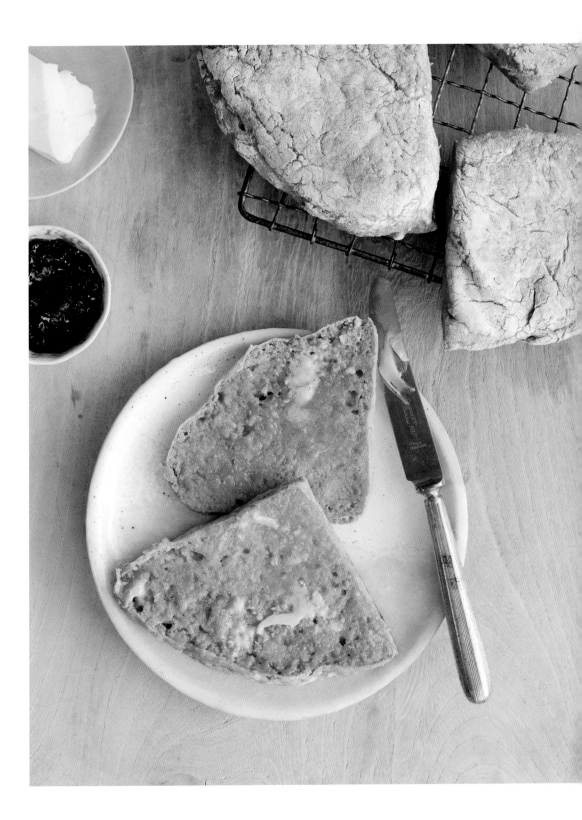

HALF-BAKED PEAR, HAZELNUT + CHOCOLATE OATMEAL

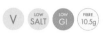

SERVES 1

My sister made a gorgeous pear, hazelnut and chocolate crumble for me, and it inspired me to make this baked oatmeal recipe. The flavours work incredibly well together.

1 pear, halved and cored

35g oats

10g flaxseed or chia seeds

½ tsp ground cinnamon

225–250ml water or milk

2 tsp honey or coconut sugar or brown sugar (optional)

5–6 hazelnuts, roughly chopped

1 square of dark chocolate, finely chopped (optional)

Preheat the oven to 180°C/350°F/gas mark 4.

Grate one half of the pear. Thinly slice the other half and set aside.

Place the grated pear in a small saucepan with the oats, flaxseed, cinnamon, water and sugar (if using). Cook over a medium heat for 3–5 minutes, until all the liquid has been absorbed.

Spoon the mixture into a small overproof dish or ramekin. Arrange the sliced pear on top, then sprinkle with the hazelnuts and chocolate (if using).

Bake for 10–15 minutes, until golden and crisp on top.

WEEKEND DINNERS

I do all my recipe developing at the weekend. I find it incredibly therapeutic to cook and bake, then serve up the results to my friends in a big banquet-style feast for everyone to dig into. I've included some dishes reminiscent of my home, including Irish Guinness Stew (see page 204) and a twist on my mum's famous Broccoli + Chicken Bake (see page 201). I've also got the perfect recipes for Sundays, when the boys come round to watch football; they love my Oat Goujons + Homemade Ketchup (see page 178) and my Mexican Loaded Sweet Potato Skins (see page 196). Of course, I don't forget those girly Saturday nights: that's when I break out my Black Bean Tostadas with Feta (see page 184).

OAT GOUJONS + HOMEMADE KETCHUP

LOW SUG · LOW SALT · LOW GI · FIBRE 4.8g

SERVES 4–6

You can make these goujons with fish or chicken, but I think they work best with cod. For me, ketchup is an essential accompaniment, but the shop-bought stuff is pretty high in sugar and salt, so I've created a lower-sugar alternative, which I promise is just as tasty.

100g cornflour

2 free-range eggs, beaten

250g oats

500g skinless cod or chicken breast, cut into 16 fingers 8 x 2cm

Vegetable oil, to fry

Salt and black pepper

Green salad, to serve

FOR THE KETCHUP

200g tomato purée

2 tbsp apple cider vinegar

2 tbsp maple syrup

100ml water

½ tsp garlic powder

½ tsp salt

Pinch of ground cinnamon

Pinch of ground allspice

First make the ketchup. Place all the ingredients in a saucepan and bring to the boil. Simmer for 5 minutes, then set aside to cool. Store in an airtight container in the fridge.

Meanwhile, place the cornflour in a bowl and mix in a teaspoon of salt and plenty of black pepper. Put the eggs and oats in 2 separate bowls. Dip each cod finger first in the flour, then the beaten egg, and finally the oats until evenly coated on all sides.

Pour a 1cm depth of vegetable oil into a pan and place over a medium–high heat. When hot, fry the cod fingers in batches for 2½–3 minutes on each side, until crisp and golden. Lift them out with a slotted spoon, drain on kitchen paper and sprinkle with salt.

Serve immediately with the ketchup and a green salad.

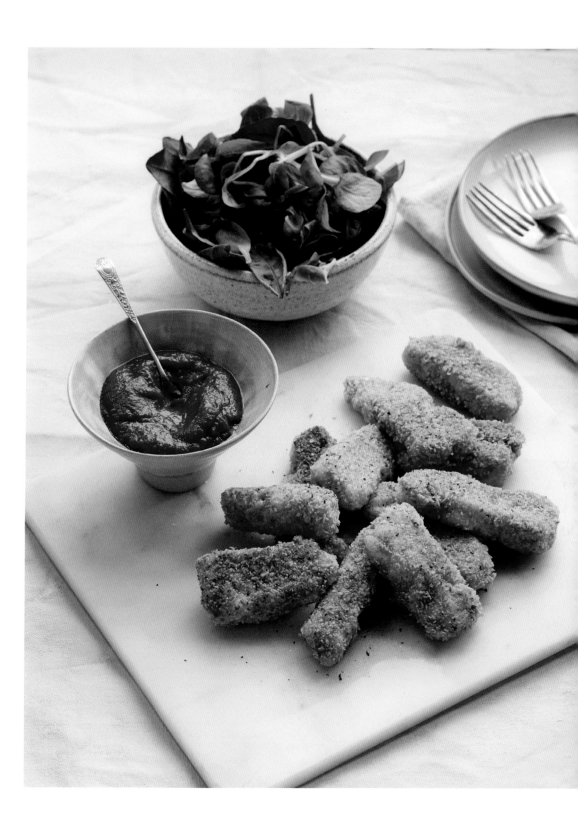

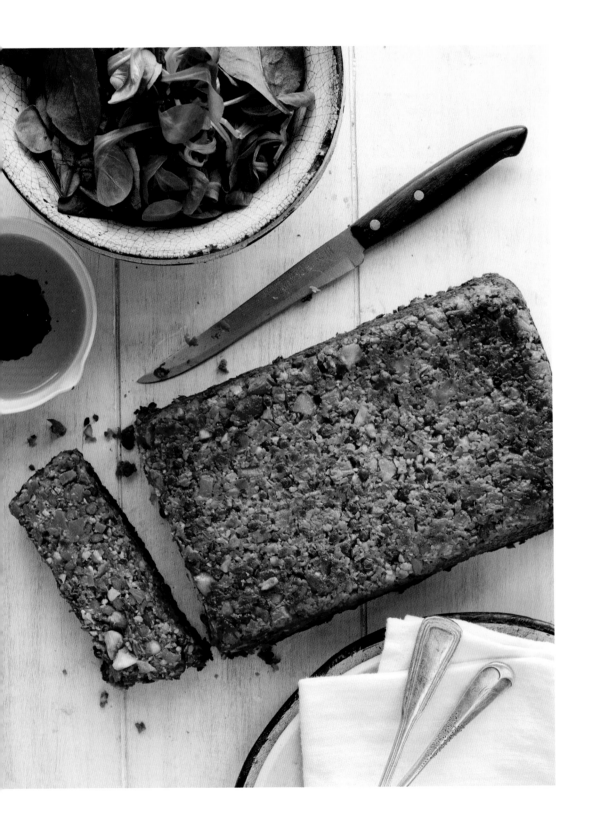

LENTIL MEATLOAF

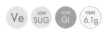

SERVES 4–6

This is the perfect Sunday roast alternative for a vegetarian or vegan, and it can be served with all the traditional side dishes. It's also a perfect picnic food in the summer.

2 tbsp olive oil

2 onions, finely chopped

1 celery stalk, finely chopped

2 carrots, peeled and finely chopped

3 garlic cloves, crushed

125g cashew nuts

150g ready-made roasted red bell peppers, drained

1 x 400g tin of green lentils, drained, or 250g cooked lentils

125g almonds, coarsely chopped

2 tbsp rosemary leaves, finely chopped

2 tbsp thyme leaves

2 tbsp tamari or dark soy sauce

Salt and black pepper

Green salad, to serve

Preheat the oven to 200°C/400°F/gas mark 6. Line a 1kg loaf tin with baking parchment.

Place the olive oil in a frying pan over a medium heat. When hot, add the onions, celery and carrot and fry for 10 minutes, until softened. Add the garlic and fry for another 2 minutes, until aromatic. Season to taste with salt and pepper, then remove from the heat.

Put half the onion mixture into a blender or food processor. Add the cashew nuts and red peppers and blitz to a rough paste. Transfer to a bowl, add the remaining onion mixture, the lentils, almonds, rosemary, thyme and tamari and mix together. Season generously with salt and pepper.

Transfer to the prepared tin, pressing it into the corners and smoothing out the surface with the back of a spoon. Bake in the oven for 1 hour, until firm and golden. Set aside to cool for 10 minutes, then turn onto a wire rack and leave to cool completely.

Serve in thick slices with a green salad.

SPINACH, MUSHROOM +
BACON QUICHE

SERVES 8–10

I love quiche – it's like breakfast and lunch and dessert all in one. It's also a great way to play around with ingredients and flavours, and to use up leftover vegetables in the fridge. For a vegetarian version, replace the bacon with sundried tomatoes, and the Gruyère with a vegetarian alternative.

250g white spelt flour

½ tsp salt

120g unsalted butter or coconut oil, chilled and cut into small pieces

2–3 tbsp water, plus extra if necessary

1 tbsp olive oil

100g smoked streaky bacon, sliced

2 onions, finely sliced

300g mushrooms, thickly sliced

150g spinach

3 free-range eggs

150ml single cream or coconut milk

3 garlic cloves, crushed

Small bunch of flat-leaf parsley, chopped

40g Gruyère cheese, grated

Salt and black pepper

Put the flour and salt into a bowl or food processor. Add the butter and rub in with your fingers, or process until the mixture resembles fine breadcrumbs. Add the water and bring together with your hands until you have a smooth ball of dough. If it is too crumbly, add a little more water just a few drops at a time, being careful not to overdo it. Flatten the dough into a thick circle, wrap it in cling film and chill for 20–30 minutes, until cold but still pliable.

Preheat the oven to 200°C/400°F/gas mark 6. Line the bottom of a 24cm tart tin with baking parchment.

Roll out the pastry between 2 sheets of floured cling film, then use to line the prepared tin. Cover and chill for 15 minutes in the fridge, or 5 minutes in the freezer. Prick the base of the pastry all over with a fork. Line the pastry case with baking parchment, fill with baking beans or rice and bake for 20 minutes. Remove the parchment and beans and bake for a further 5 minutes.

Meanwhile, put the oil in a frying pan over a medium–high heat. When hot, add the bacon, onions and mushrooms and fry for 6–8 minutes, until the bacon and mushrooms are golden and the onions have softened. Add the spinach and stir until wilted. Remove from the heat and drain off any vegetable liquid (this can be saved for use in soups and stews).

Put the eggs into a large bowl, add the cream, garlic and most of the parsley and season well with salt and pepper. Pour into the baked pastry case and top with the bacon mixture and the cheese. Cover with foil and bake for 20 minutes. Remove the foil and bake for a further 15–20 minutes, until golden and set. Top with the remaining parsley and serve immediately.

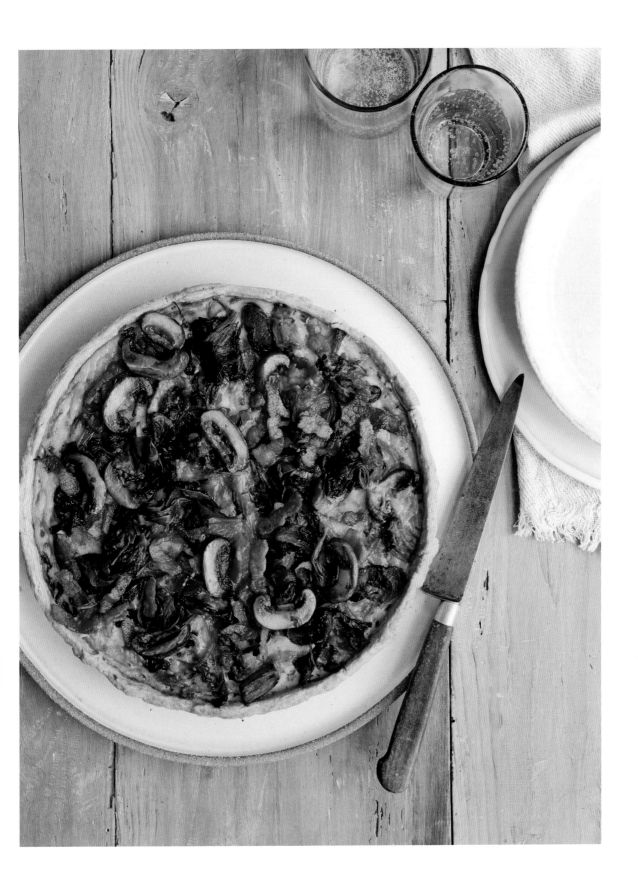

BLACK BEAN TOSTADAS WITH FETA

SERVES 3–4

This recipe was a bit of an experiment when I had the girls over for dinner one Friday night. To make the tostadas I cut circles out of ready-made tortillas using the rim of a pint glass – could I be any more Irish? They worked really well and everyone loved digging in and adding their own toppings.

8 corn tortillas

1 tbsp olive oil

2 garlic cloves, grated

½ white onion, diced

½ tsp cayenne pepper

½ tsp ground cumin

2 x 400g tins of red kidney beans or black beans, drained and rinsed

100–150ml water

Salt

TO SERVE

100g feta cheese, crumbled

Pickled Red Onion (see page 94)

Fresh coriander leaves

Jalapeño chillies, deseeded and sliced

Avocado slices

Cherry tomatoes, halved

Preheat the oven to 200°C/400°F/gas mark 6.

Using a 9cm pastry cutter or the rim of a similar-sized tumbler, cut 3–4 circles out of each tortilla. Place them on a baking tray and bake for 5 minutes, then turn them over and bake for a further 4–5 minutes, until crisp and light brown. Alternatively, you can fry the tostadas in hot olive oil until golden on each side. Keep warm in tinfoil while you cook the beans.

Heat the olive oil in a large frying pan. When hot, add the garlic and onion, and fry for 2 minutes, until soft. Stir in the cayenne, cumin and some salt.

Add the beans and the water, and cook until the beans are tender, about 5 minutes. Using a potato masher or the back of a wooden spoon, roughly mash the beans. Cook for another minute, then add salt to taste. Transfer to a serving bowl.

Serve the tostadas with the mashed beans and bowls of toppings for everyone to pick and mix their own combinations.

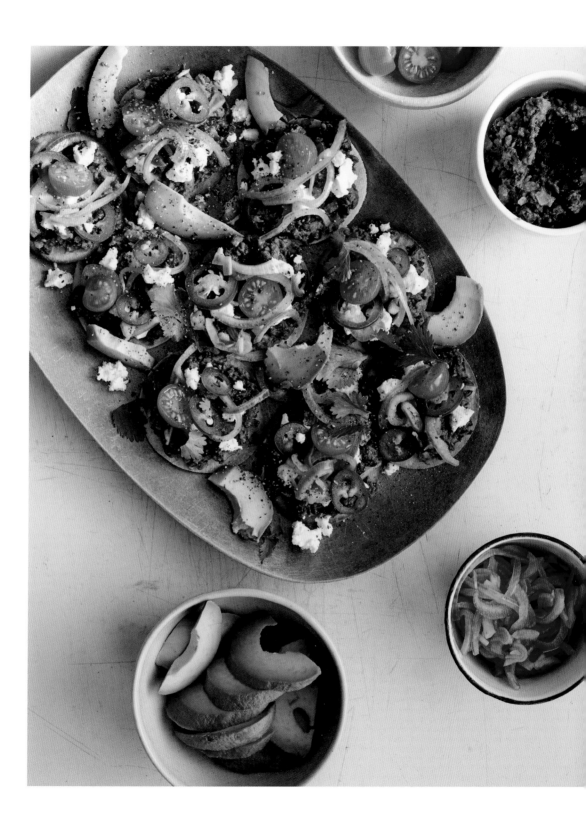

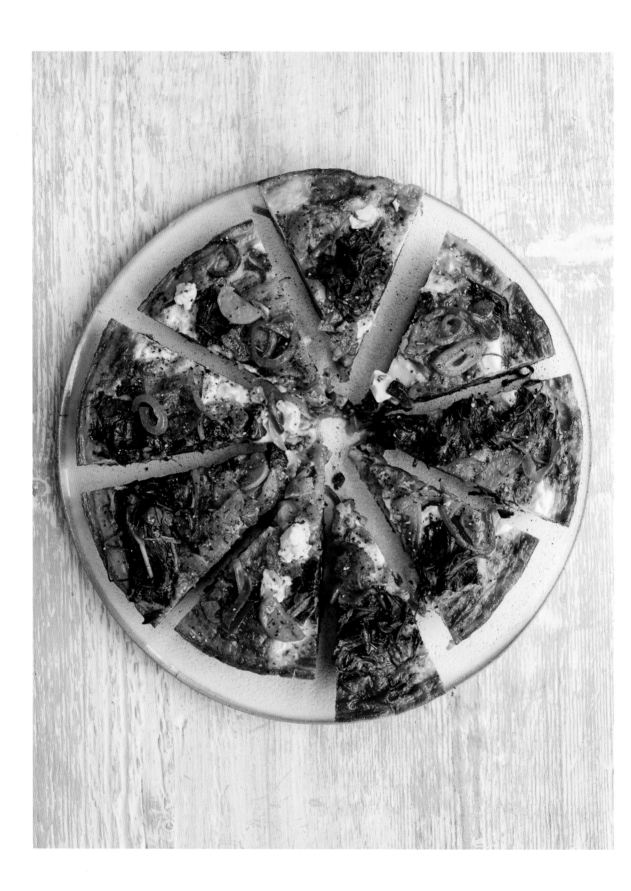

SWEET POTATO FRITTATA

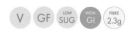

SERVES 6-8

This frittata is so impressive when it's cut because of all the gorgeous layers of sweet potato and spinach. One frittata feeds a big crowd, and if you have any leftovers (highly unlikely) it's lovely cold the next day for breakfast or lunch.

4 tbsp olive oil

1 red onion, halved and
    sliced into semicircles

1 garlic clove, grated

2 sweet potatoes (about
    450g in total), peeled
    and finely sliced
    widthways

1 tsp dried basil

1 tsp dried oregano

½ tsp salt and pepper

2-3 handfuls of spinach

8 free-range eggs

75ml milk

100g feta cheese

Preheat the oven to 200°C/400°F/gas mark 6.

Heat the olive oil in a large frying pan. When hot, fry the onion and garlic over a medium heat until soft, about 3–5 minutes.

Add the sweet potato slices, dried herbs and salt. Cook for 10 minutes, stirring now and then, until the potatoes have softened and browned.

When the potatoes are done, toss in the spinach and cook until wilted. This will take just a minute or so. Remove from the heat and set aside.

Whisk the eggs and milk together in a bowl and season with salt and pepper. Pour into a 20cm ovenproof frying pan or casserole dish. Add the vegetables, ensuring they are visible, then crumble the feta on top.

Bake for 35–40 minutes, until golden and cooked right through. Set aside to cool a little before slicing.

SUNDAY ROAST CHICKEN
+ ROASTED VEGETABLES

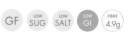

SERVES 4–5

Cooking a roast for a crowd can be slightly daunting, but this one-pot recipe takes at least some of the stress away. Serve it with Sweet Potato Gratin (see pages 190–191) and you're bound to impress your friends and family.

1 whole chicken
(about 1.5kg)

Zest and juice 1 lemon

2 tbsp olive oil

4–5 sprigs of thyme,
leaves roughly chopped

300g carrots, peeled
and cut into chunks

300g parsnips, peeled
and cut into long batons

2 red onions, cut into
wedges

1 head of garlic, cloves
separated and peeled

Salt and black pepper

Preheat the oven to 200°C/400°F/gas mark 6.

Put the chicken in a large roasting tin and squeeze the lemon juice over it. Rub in 1 tablespoon of the oil, then sprinkle with the thyme and plenty of seasoning. Roast for 30 minutes.

Put the carrots, parsnips and onions in a bowl, add the remaining tablespoon of oil, the lemon zest and plenty of black pepper and toss together.

Transfer the chicken to a plate. Scatter the vegetables into the roasting tin, arranging the garlic cloves around the middle, then put the chicken on top. Return to the oven for a further 45 minutes, tossing the veg after 20 minutes.

When the chicken is cooked and the vegetables are tender and lightly browned, transfer the bird to a serving platter. Cover with foil and set aside to rest for 10 minutes.

Scatter the vegetables around the chicken and serve with the Sweet Potato Gratin (see opposite page).

SWEET POTATO GRATIN

SERVES 4–5

It was always a treat when Mum made potato gratin for Sunday dinner. I've added a twist to her version by using sweet potato and coconut cream, but you could use regular white spuds if you prefer. One thing to note is that sweet potato gets a lot softer than regular potato, and holds its shape less well, but the flavour is yummy.

2 tbsp olive oil

1 onion, finely chopped

4 garlic cloves, crushed

2 tbsp thyme leaves, plus extra to sprinkle

2 tbsp rosemary leaves, finely chopped

75ml chicken or vegetable stock

100ml coconut cream

800g sweet potatoes, washed, dried and very thinly sliced

2 tbsp freshly grated Parmesan cheese

Salt and black pepper

Preheat the oven to 200°C/400°F/gas mark 6. Set out a 20 x 26cm ovenproof baking dish.

Put the oil in a frying pan over a medium heat. When hot, add the onion and fry for 8 minutes, until softened. Add the garlic, thyme and rosemary and fry for another 2 minutes, until aromatic. Pour in the stock and coconut cream, bring to the boil, then simmer for 1 minute. Remove from the heat.

Place a layer of the sweet potato slices in the bottom of the baking dish. Season lightly and drizzle over a few spoonfuls of the stock. Continue layering the sweet potato, lightly seasoning and adding stock as you go, until everything is used up. Cover the dish with tinfoil, making sure it is very well sealed to prevent steam from escaping. Bake for 45 minutes, until the potato is soft.

Remove the foil, sprinkle over the Parmesan and a little extra thyme, then return to the oven for 15 minutes, until golden on top. Serve immediately.

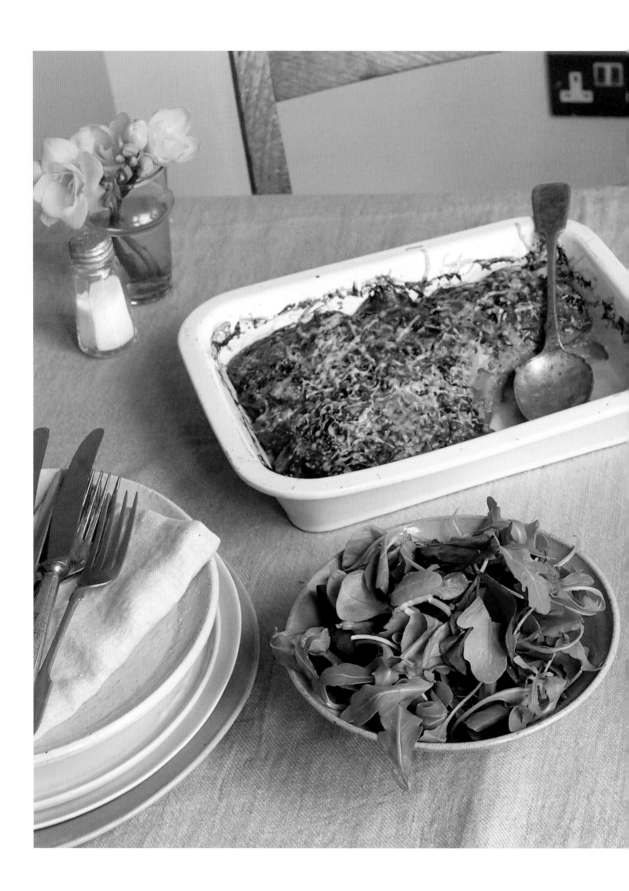

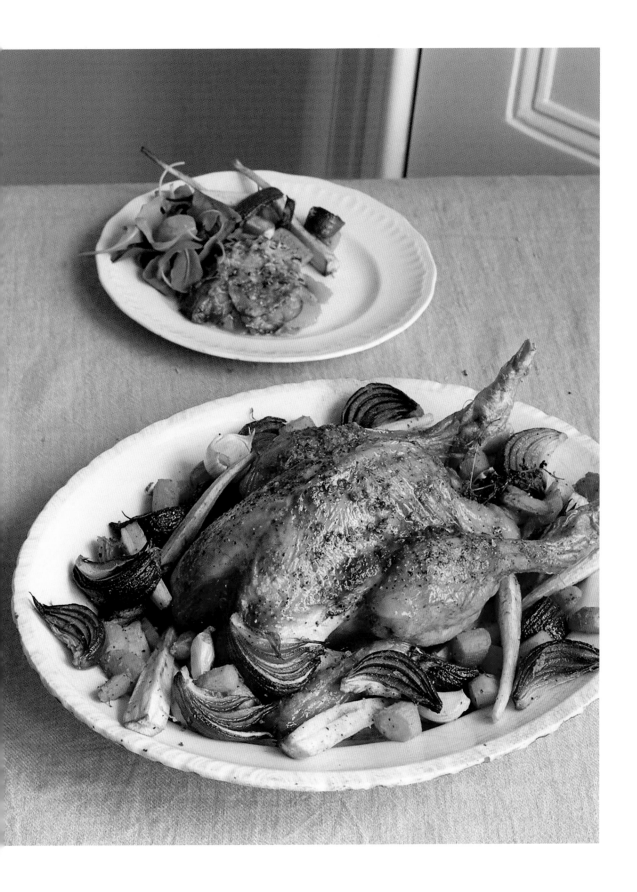

MINDFULNESS

Let's start with the basics. What exactly is mindfulness?

There are plenty of definitions out there. My personal favourite is that of Dr Jon Kabat-Zinn, one of the most famous practitioners in mindfulness meditation, who describes mindfulness as 'Paying attention in a particular way: on purpose, in the present moment, and non-judgmentally'.

This definition can be broken down into three key elements:

1. ON PURPOSE

Mindfulness involves consciously directing your awareness. It means having the intention of staying with your experience, whether that means following your breath or focusing on the texture of food in your mouth. Regardless of technique, you are actively engaged. Your intention is in the here and now.

2. IN THE PRESENT

It is normal for the mind to get distracted and lost in thought. Mindfulness is not, as some may think, the practice of emptying the mind, but of noticing when the mind wanders, and of returning, again and again, to the present moment.

3. WITHOUT JUDGING

It is human instinct to judge things as good or bad, right or wrong. When you are mindful and notice judgements arise, make a mental note of them and let them pass.

In simple terms, mindfulness is actively noticing things; for instance, how your ribcage expands like an accordion when you breathe in and out, or how the light of a candle flickers from a draught in the room. The thing is, mindfulness is a skill we all naturally possess, but if we don't practise it, we find it more difficult to do. Using the analogy of building muscle, if we don't use it, we lose it, so if we don't train our mindfulness muscle, it won't exist or grow. The more we use it, the more we can strengthen our ability to detach ourselves from mental distractions and develop a reflective mind. We can switch off autopilot and live – really live.

HOW DOES MINDFULNESS WORK?

It's remarkable but true that part of the nervous system – the parasympathetic nervous system (PNS) – exists purely for us to feel peaceful and calm. Its cousin is the sympathetic nervous system (SNS), which has the opposite job of getting you fired up to fight or flee when you need to. Both the PNS and SNS are part of the autonomic nervous system, which controls all the tasks that your body performs without any conscious thought, including breathing, digestion and the production of hormones.

From an evolutionary standpoint, the primary role of the SNS is to keep us safe from danger. Obviously, the dangers we avoid nowadays aren't exactly the same as those of our ancestors; running from your boss doesn't quite compare to running from a lion, but it's the same principle. Activation of the SNS raises the heart rate, increases the breathing, releases stress hormones and shunts blood away from the digestive tract to the muscles so that we have the energy to escape (or stand frozen like a rabbit in the headlights). Once we are out of danger, the PNS kicks in and slows the breathing and heart rate, moves blood back to the digestive system and repairs the hormonal chaos that the SNS caused.

These systems work in the background all the time. For example, when you stand up from lying down, your SNS acts to constrict your blood vessels, preventing your blood pressure from dropping which could leave you flat on the floor. Activating the SNS is no bad thing, but we really do live in a time of SNS gone amok when, more often than not, we are in a state of stress.

Although the system is technically out of our control, we can manipulate it to some extent through breathing techniques, mindfulness and meditation.

How about we give it a go, right here, right now?

You can activate the parasympathetic nervous system through a simple breathing exercise that incorporates visualising the sides of a square, each side representing a count of four.

SQUARE BREATHING TECHNIQUE

First of all, I want you to sit up tall in a chair and plant your feet on the ground (if you're in bed, prop some pillows behind your back). Try to keep your back as straight as you can so that you're not slumped and can fully expand your ribcage. Your hands can lie open or gently clasped in your lap. Use any four-sided object in the room as a visual guide (window, picture frame, post-it note or computer screen) or visualise one in your head. Relax your gaze or close your eyes.

- Take a deep breath in through your nostrils for four seconds, really filling your lungs.

- Hold the breath for 4...3....2...1

- Exhale through your nose to the count of 4...3...2...1

- And hold for 4...3...2...1

This is one cycle, but you can do it as many times as you feel necessary. I'm not ashamed to say that I've often locked myself in the toilet on the hospital ward to practise this once or twice when I can feel the stress beginning to rise inside me. It always brings me back to a calmer state and allows me to think more clearly.

MINDFULNESS IN THE NHS

As doctors, we are beginning to integrate mindfulness more and more into our practice, and I couldn't be more excited. In the UK, the government's National Institute for Health and Clinical Excellence (NICE) recommends Mindfulness-Based Cognitive Therapy (MBCT) in their guidelines for management of recurrent depression (i.e.

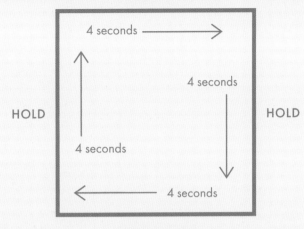

three or more episodes of depression). In studies it has been shown to significantly reduce the risk of relapse of recurrent depression compared to the usual treatment or controls. MBCT helps those who suffer with recurrent depression by teaching them to recognise the negative thoughts, feelings and beliefs that can easily spiral into a depressive relapse and to respond constructively.

So far, mindfulness is only creeping its way into conventional medicine, so don't be surprised if your GP isn't up to speed with it yet. There is an evidence base behind it but, to be honest, not everything needs a wealth of scientific papers to be life-changing. What's to be lost by trying something that is non-invasive, has no side-effects and can be practised at home for free? I would never ask you to self-treat when you are unwell, but I hope that these simple techniques will enable you to live your life a little more stress-free and to visit your GP less often.

Your mind just slows down, and you see a tremendous expanse in the moment. You see so much more than you could see before. It's a discipline; you have to practise it.

- Steve Jobs, former head of Apple Inc.

MEDITATION VS MINDFULNESS

Many people get confused between meditation and mindfulness, and it's no surprise because they do cross over in several ways. I'll try to try explain as best I can how they differ. The main difference is that mindfulness is slightly more of an informal practice in which you're attempting to be more aware of everything as you go about your daily life. Meditation requires actively taking time out from normal day-to-day activities in order to practise it, and to focus your attention on connecting with yourself.

Often when I speak to people about meditation they tell me that they can't do it because they 'can't clear their minds', so they become frustrated and give up. I can completely relate to this, and it was one of my reasons for initially having so much resistance to meditation and mindfulness. It is a common frustration, but it is based on a common misconception – that we are supposed to be clearing our minds. There are many forms of meditation, but the most popular form in the western world is mindfulness meditation, which originates from the teachings of Buddhism. The object of mindfulness meditation is not to clear the mind of thoughts (although sometimes that does happen), but to observe your thoughts as they arise and gently bring your attention back to your breathing.

There are several aspects to this technique, and many people practise it in their own unique way, but the following elements are usually included:

- A quiet location with minimal distractions

- A comfortable seated position

- A focus of attention, generally the breath

- An open mind, allowing distractions and thoughts to come and go naturally without judging them

If you are completely new to meditation and are unsure how to start practising, I would recommend trying guided meditation as part of a group or class, watching a YouTube video, listening to a podcast, or using an app such as Calm or Headspace. It's much easier to understand what the whole meditating business is about when someone talks you through it step-by-step (they also tend to play really relaxing spa music, which helps).

If you just sit and observe, you will see how restless your mind is. If you try to calm it, that initially makes things worse. Over time, though, it does calm, and when it does, there's room to hear more subtle things – that's when your intuition starts to blossom, you start to see things more clearly and are more in the present.

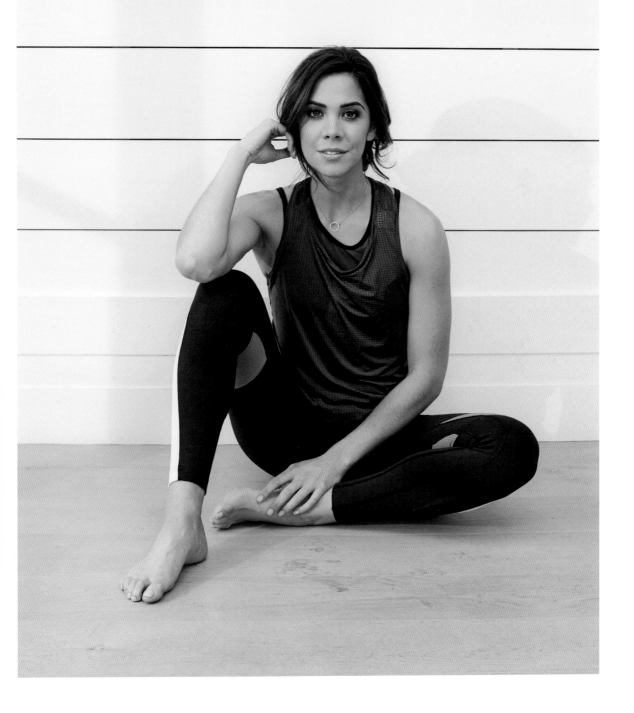

MEXICAN LOADED SWEET POTATO SKINS

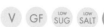

SERVES 4 AS A MAIN, OR 8 AS A SIDE

If I had to eat one cuisine for the rest of my life, it would probably be Mexican. It's always my top choice for celebrating a special occasion so that I can get loaded nachos and a good margarita. This recipe is slightly more virtuous than what you get in restaurants, but feel free to serve it up with margaritas nevertheless. While great as a main, it also makes a good side dish with chicken, fish or steak.

4 sweet potatoes, washed and dried

1 tbsp olive oil, plus extra to rub

1 small red onion, diced

2 garlic cloves, grated

1 x 400g tin of red kidney beans, drained and rinsed

1 small tin of sweetcorn (about 150g), drained

1 red chilli, deseeded and finely chopped

Juice of 1 lime

1 tsp smoked paprika

1 tsp ground cumin

4 tbsp grated Cheddar cheese (optional)

Salt and black pepper

Preheat the oven to 180°C/350°F/gas mark 4.

Rub the sweet potatoes with a little olive oil, then slice them in half lengthways. Place in a baking tray, cut-side up, and roast for 45–50 minutes, until fork-tender and the skins are coming away from the flesh. Set aside to cool for 5 minutes.

Holding a halved sweet potato in a tea towel, use a spoon to scoop most of the flesh into a large bowl – you want to leave a thin 'wall' of flesh inside the skin for support. Repeat with each half, then mash the sweet potato in the bowl.

Heat the tablespoon of oil in a frying pan. When hot, fry the onion and garlic over a medium heat for 5 minutes, until soft and translucent.

Add the onion and garlic to the mashed potato, along with the kidney beans, corn, chilli, lime juice, spices and little seasoning. Mix well.

Scoop the potato mixture back into the skins, top with the cheese (if using) and pop back in the oven for 10 more minutes.

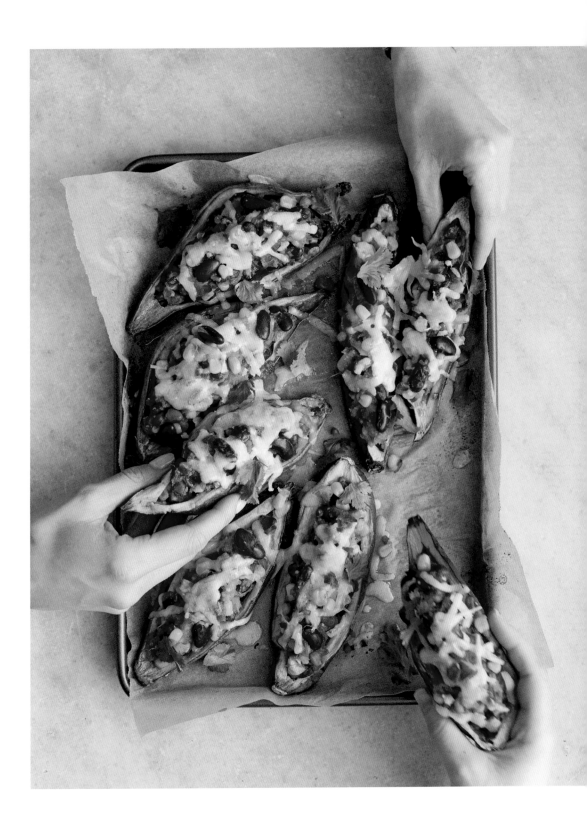

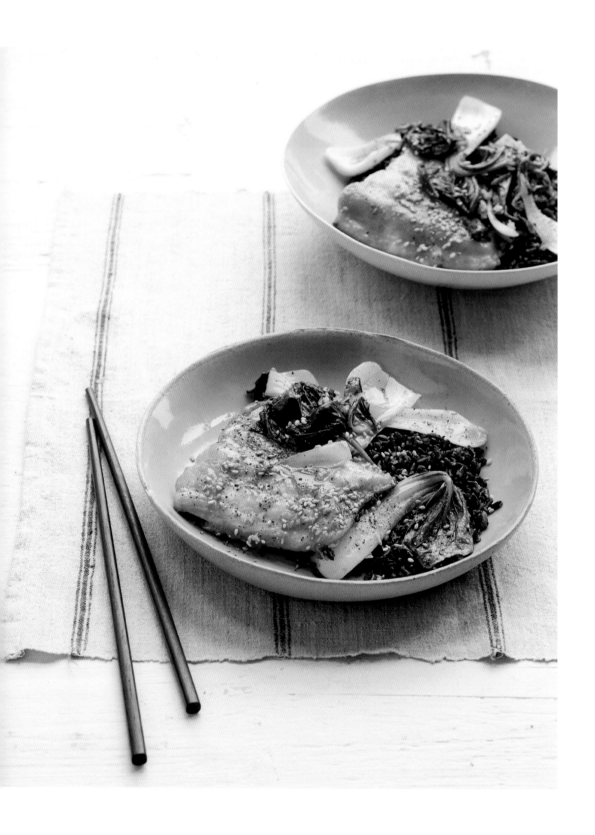

MISO SALMON, BLACK RICE + ASIAN GREENS

SERVES 2

Miso is a traditional Japanese food made from fermented soya beans, rice or grain and salt. It might sound a bit strange if you've never tried it, but it adds the most amazing, intense flavour to this simple salmon recipe and it's something I always have in my fridge. You can find miso in the Japanese section of most large supermarkets.

2 tbsp white miso paste

2 tsp soy sauce

1 tbsp maple syrup

2 salmon fillets

125g black rice

250ml water

1 tbsp sesame seed oil, plus extra to drizzle

1 garlic clove, chopped

1 head of pak choi, quartered lengthways

2 handfuls of spinach

1 tbsp sesame seeds

Salt

Combine the miso paste, soy sauce and maple syrup in a bowl. Coat the salmon fillets in the mixture, then cover with cling film and marinate in the fridge overnight, or for at least 2 hours.

Put the rice in a saucepan with the water and a pinch of salt. Bring to the boil, then cover and simmer for 40–45 minutes, stirring occasionally. Drain.

While the rice is cooking, preheat the oven to 200°C/400°F/gas mark 6. Line a roasting tray with tinfoil.

Place the salmon in the prepared tray and roast for 15 minutes, until the flesh flakes easily and is cooked through.

Place a wok or frying pan on a medium–high heat. Add the tablespoon of sesame oil and fry the garlic for 30 seconds, or until just beginning to sizzle.

Add the pak choi and 1 tablespoon of water and stir-fry for 1–2 minutes. Add the spinach and stir–fry for 1–2 minutes, until just wilted.

Serve the greens with the salmon, adding a drizzle of sesame oil and a sprinkling of sesame seeds.

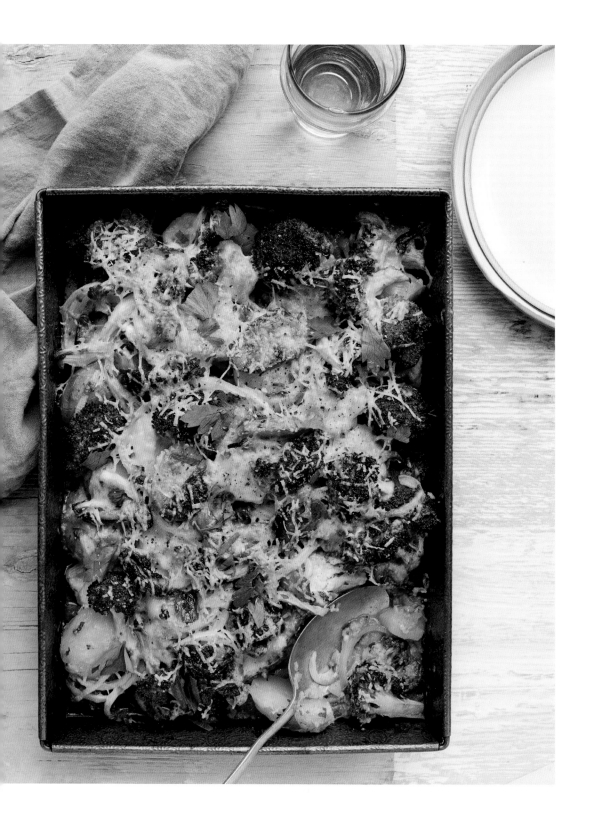

BROCCOLI + CHICKEN BAKE

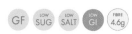

SERVES 6

My mum used to make this with a creamy sauce, topping the broccoli and chicken mixture with thinly sliced potatoes, Parmesan and Tayto crisps. Now Tayto crisps are essentially a staple food in Ireland, so if you have never tried them, get yourself over there and pick up a packet of cheese and onion from the nearest newsagent. Trust me on this one. I've left crisps out of this recipe, but I will make no judgement if you wish to use them.

500g potatoes, peeled and roughly chopped

1 tbsp olive oil

2 skinless chicken breasts, cut into bite-sized chunks

200g mushrooms, thickly sliced

300g broccoli, broken into florets

1 onion, sliced

4 garlic cloves, crushed

250g crème fraîche

150g mature Cheddar cheese

2 tsp Dijon mustard

Large handful of flat-leaf parsley, finely chopped, plus extra to sprinkle

2 tbsp freshly grated Parmesan cheese

Salt and black pepper

Preheat the oven to 200°C/400°F/gas mark 6.

Put the potatoes into a pan of salted water, bring to the boil, then simmer for 5 minutes. Drain and set aside.

Meanwhile, put the oil into a frying pan over a medium–high heat. When hot, add the chicken and mushrooms and fry for 8–10 minutes, until the chicken is cooked through and the mushrooms are golden.

Transfer the chicken mixture to a bowl and combine with all the remaining ingredients, except the Parmesan. Tip into a large, ovenproof baking dish, cover with tinfoil and bake for 30 minutes.

Remove the foil, scatter over the Parmesan and continue to cook for 15 minutes, until golden on top. Sprinkle with extra parsley and serve immediately.

SWEET + SMOKY CHICKPEA-STUFFED SWEET POTATOES

SERVES 2-3, DEPENDING ON APPETITE

There are few combinations better than chickpeas and tahini, but team them with soft, almost mushy sweet potatoes and you're really onto a winner.

3 sweet potatoes, washed and dried

1 tbsp olive oil, plus extra for rubbing

1 x 400g tin of chickpeas, drained and rinsed

1 garlic clove, grated

½ tsp ground cumin

½ tsp ground cinnamon

½ tsp smoked paprika

1 red bell pepper, deseeded and diced

1 lime, halved

2 tbsp tahini

1 tbsp maple syrup

2-3 tbsp water

Salt

TO SERVE

Spring onion, chopped

Lime wedges

Fresh spinach

Olive oil

Preheat the oven to 200°C/400°F/gas mark 6. Line a roasting tray with tinfoil.

Cut the potatoes in half lengthways, then rub each half with a little olive oil and salt. Place in the prepared tray, flesh-side down, and bake for 35–40 minutes, until soft right through.

Meanwhile, put the chickpeas in a bowl and add the garlic, cumin, cinnamon, paprika, red pepper and the juice of half the lime. Mix well.

Place the tablespoon of olive oil in a large frying pan over a medium heat. When hot, add the chickpea mixture and fry for about 5 minutes, until hot and toasted.

Put the tahini in a small bowl, add the maple syrup, the juice from the remaining lime and the water. Whisk together until smooth, adding extra water if necessary to make it a pouring consistency.

Spoon the chickpea mixture over the baked sweet potatoes, drizzle with the tahini sauce and top with spring onions. Serve with lime wedges and some fresh spinach leaves, dressed with olive oil.

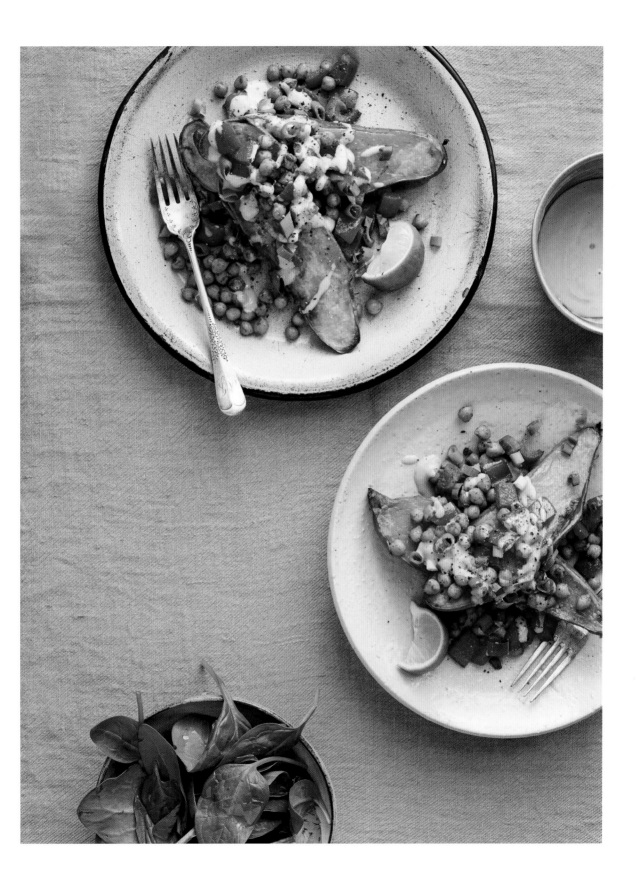

IRISH GUINNESS STEW

SERVES 4

Well, you didn't think I was going to leave out Guinness, now, did you? It's an old wives' tale in Ireland that pregnant women should drink Guinness because it's a good source of iron. I had a look into this and, sadly, it doesn't seem like there is enough iron in a pint of Guinness to make much of a contribution to dietary requirements. Added to that, it's not a good idea to drink alcohol during pregnancy. Dubious health benefits aside, Guinness does taste great in stews, leaving the meat lovely and tender.

3 tbsp olive oil

500g beef shoulder
   or stewing beef, cut
   into chunks

2 onions, chopped

3 carrots, peeled and
   roughly chopped

300g potatoes, peeled
   and chopped into
   3cm chunks

2 celery stalks, chopped

3 garlic cloves, crushed

2 tbsp cornflour

300ml beef stock

500ml Guinness

2 bay leaves

Salt and black pepper

Put 2 tablespoons of the oil into a large flameproof casserole dish over a high heat. Once hot, add the beef and fry for 3–5 minutes, until browned. Season and set aside on a plate.

Add the remaining tablespoon of oil to the empty dish, then add the onions, carrots, potatoes and celery and fry for 5 minutes. Add the garlic and fry for 2 more minutes, until aromatic.

Put the cornflour into a mug or bowl, add a little of the stock and stir until dissolved. Pour into the casserole dish with the remaining stock, the Guinness, bay leaves, reserved beef and salt to taste (take care with the seasoning if your stock already contains salt). Bring to the boil, then simmer, uncovered, for 45–50 minutes, until the meat is tender and the liquid has reduced and thickened.

Serve with crusty bread.

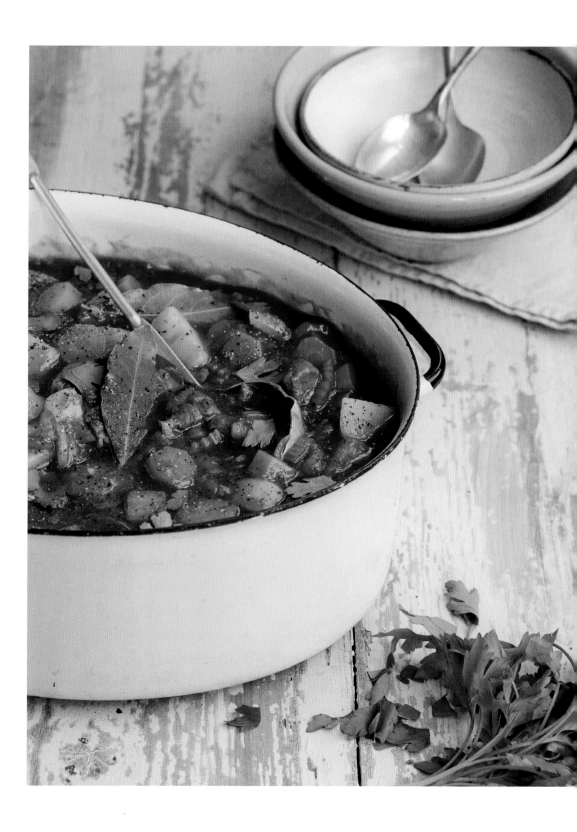

BAKED AUBERGINE WITH TOMATOES + MOZZARELLA

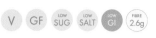

SERVES 4

My first book featured a sticky soy-roasted aubergine, and it pretty much became the star of the book – everyone loved it! However, many people I come across dislike aubergine, which I think is largely because it is often poorly cooked, so it tastes watery, rubbery and slimy. Roasting aubergine dries it out, so it's less likely to hold water, and the balsamic marinade adds a wonderful sweetness to the vegetable. This dish is great as a vegetarian main course served with couscous or crushed baby potatoes, or gorgeous as a side with fish.

2 tbsp olive oil

2 tbsp balsamic vinegar

2 garlic cloves, grated

2 aubergines, halved
   lengthways

1 mozzarella ball

2 tomatoes

Handful of pine nuts

Salt

Fresh basil leaves,
   to garnish

Heat the oven to 220°C/450°F/gas mark 8. Line a baking sheet with tinfoil.

Put the oil, vinegar and garlic in a bowl and whisk together.

Score the flesh of each aubergine half in a criss-cross pattern. Spoon the marinade evenly over each aubergine half, ensuring it is well coated and the marinade is absorbed deep into the flesh. Transfer to a roasting tin, flesh-side up. Sprinkle with a little salt and pour any remaining marinade over the top.

Roast for 30–35 minutes, until softened. When done, they should be soft to the point of a knife.

Meanwhile, slice the mozzarella and tomatoes very thinly.

Once the aubergine is cooked, arrange the slices of tomato and cheese on top of each half and sprinkle with some pine nuts. Return to oven for another 5–10 minutes, or until the cheese has melted and the pine nuts are a shade darker (taking care not to let them burn).

Garnish with the basil leaves before serving.

NOURISHING BAKES
+ SWEETS

Bread . . . fresh from the oven . . . still warm . . . butter slightly melting . . . and a dollop of sweet jam . . . are there many better things in life? I'm not so sure.

I love to bake, perhaps even more than I love to cook, but there is definitely a bit more skill required. I can't really whack a whole load of ingredients together and hope for the best as I do with soups and stews. Instead, I have to be more calculated and mindful. This instantly forces me to slow down and switch off from the busy world outside and inside my head, and allows me to be present in the moment. It lets my hands do the work and my mind become quiet.

Of course, the primary point of food is to sustain us and keep us alive, but it's also hugely important that we enjoy our food and take pleasure in the act of preparing it. I hope this section will help you to find some peace in your busy world.

PORRIDGE BREAD

**MAKES A
900G LOAF
(10 SLICES)**

Everyone loves freshly baked bread, but not many people like the lengthy process that it often involves. Personally, I love to bake bread. I find it very therapeutic, but I don't always have time to do it. This recipe is not your typical bread recipe as the base is oats and yogurt, but the end result will amaze you. Porridge bread is widely made in Ireland, but I've tweaked the recipe over the past few years and I think (think) I've nailed it. For a low-sugar version omit the dried fruit.

Butter or coconut oil,
   to grease

1 flax egg (see tip below)

300g oats, plus extra to
   sprinkle

1 tsp bicarbonate of soda

½ tsp salt

1 tsp ground cinnamon

60g dried fruit, chopped
   (I like a mixture of
   apricots, dates and
   raisins)

60g mixed seeds, plus extra
   to sprinkle (I used half
   pumpkin, half sunflower)

1 x 500ml tub of natural
   yogurt

1 tbsp treacle or blackstrap
   molasses

Preheat the oven to 200°C/400°F/gas mark 6. Grease a 900g loaf tin, or line it with baking parchment.

Prepare the flax egg. Meanwhile, put the oats in a large bowl and mix in the bicarbonate of soda, salt, cinnamon, dried fruit and seeds.

Add the yogurt and treacle to the flax egg mixture and stir until combined. Tip into the bowl of dry ingredients and mix well.

Pour the mixture into the prepared tin and sprinkle with some extra oats and seeds. Bake for 25 minutes, then lower the temperature to 160°C/325°F/gas mark 3, cover the loaf with tinfoil and bake for a further 30 minutes, or until a skewer inserted in the centre comes out clean.

Allow to cool for 15 minutes in the tin before transferring to a wire rack to cool for a further 1–2 hours before slicing.

TIP: *To make a flax egg (a good substitute in many baking recipes for a regular egg), place 1½ tbsp ground flaxseed and 3 tbsp water in a small bowl. Set aside to soak for 5 minutes, until thickened and set.*

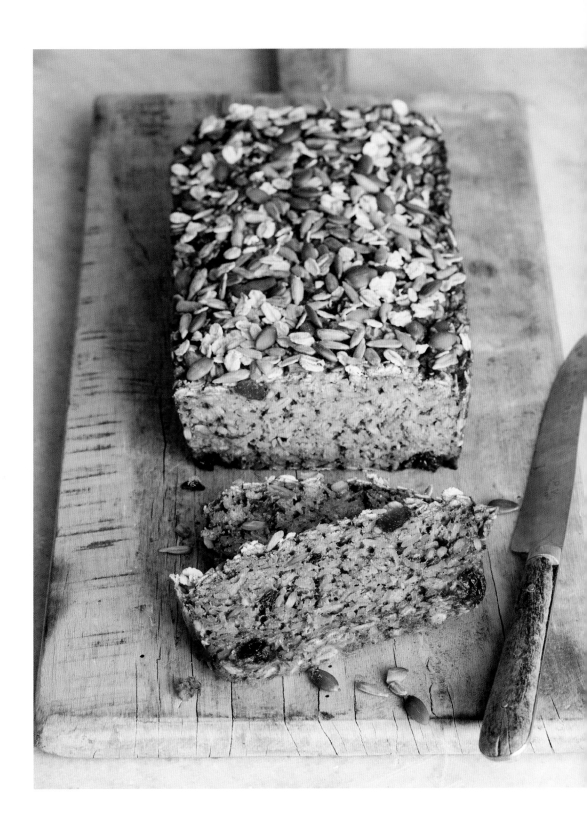

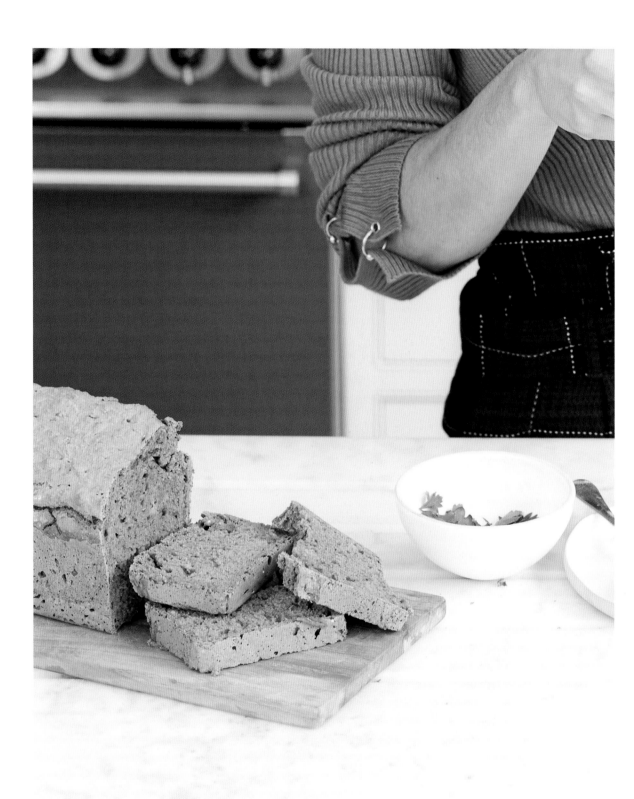

RYE BREAD

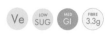

**MAKES A
450G LOAF
(10 SLICES)**

When I was nineteen, I had a lot of digestive issues and was diagnosed with irritable bowel syndrome (IBS). Bread, particularly the white bagels and baguettes I was eating, seemed to trigger my symptoms, so I cut them out of my diet, and for a long time I didn't eat bread at all. Eventually , I felt like I was massively missing out on one of my favourite foods, so I started to experiment with making breads made from non-wheat flours and from spelt, which is a form of wheat but relatively low in gluten. I don't have any problem tolerating bread now, so either I misinterpreted my triggers, or my changes paid off. Rye bread is one of my favourites, particularly served with salmon and cream cheese.

Coconut oil, to grease
300g wholegrain rye flour
200g white spelt flour
1 tsp baking powder
1 tsp bicarbonate of soda
1 tsp salt
2 tbsp blackstrap molasses
560ml tepid water

Preheat the oven to 180°C/350°F/gas mark 4. Grease a 450g loaf tin and line it with baking parchment.

Mix all the dry ingredients together in a bowl.

In a separate bowl, combine the molasses and water, stirring until the molasses has dissolved. Add this liquid to the dry ingredients and mix well.

Pour the mixture into the prepared tin and bake for 50 minutes, until well risen and 'set'. Remove from the tin and return the loaf to the oven for 15 minutes, until it has a firm golden crust. Set aside on a wire rack to cool before serving.

COURGETTE + WALNUT LOAF

**MAKES A
900G LOAF
(10 SLICES)**

Isn't it funny how the folds and wrinkles of walnuts resemble the human brain? That, combined with their high content of omega 3 fatty acids, makes it no wonder they're called 'brain food'. All that goodness is packed into this recipe, which is actually something between a loaf and a cake. As it's not very sweet, it can be served with soup, or toasted and eaten with eggs, but it's also gorgeous with butter and jam – and a cup of tea, of course!

80ml rapeseed oil or
   melted coconut oil, plus
   extra to grease
120g courgette
2 free-range eggs
80g honey or maple syrup
100ml milk
250g spelt flour
½ tsp salt
1 tsp baking powder
½ tsp bicarbonate of soda
Handful of chopped
   walnuts

Preheat the oven to 200°C/400°F/gas mark 6. Grease a 900g loaf tin and line it with baking parchment.

Grate the courgette, then wrap it in kitchen paper or a clean tea towel and squeeze out the excess moisture.

Break the eggs into a bowl and beat them together. Add the oil, honey and milk and whisk to combine.

Place the flour in a separate bowl and stir in the salt, baking powder and bicarbonate of soda. Add the egg mixture, courgette and nuts and mix well.

Pour the mixture into the prepared tin and bake for 45–50 minutes, or until a skewer inserted in the centre comes out clean.

Set the loaf aside to cool in the tin for 10 minutes, then turn it onto a wire rack to cool for 30 minutes before slicing.

The loaf is moist, so will keep for 2–3 days in a bread bin, or for up to 5 days in an airtight plastic container in the fridge. It can also be sliced and frozen for up to 3 months.

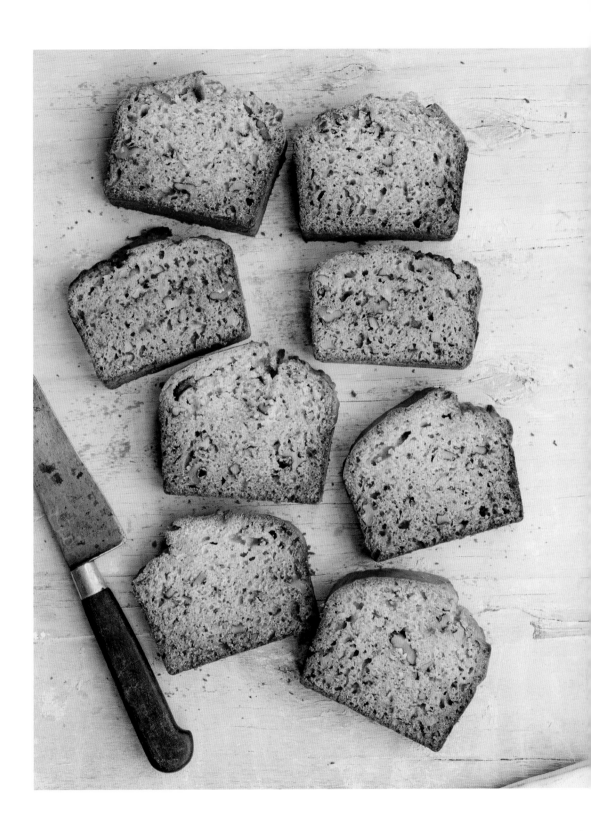

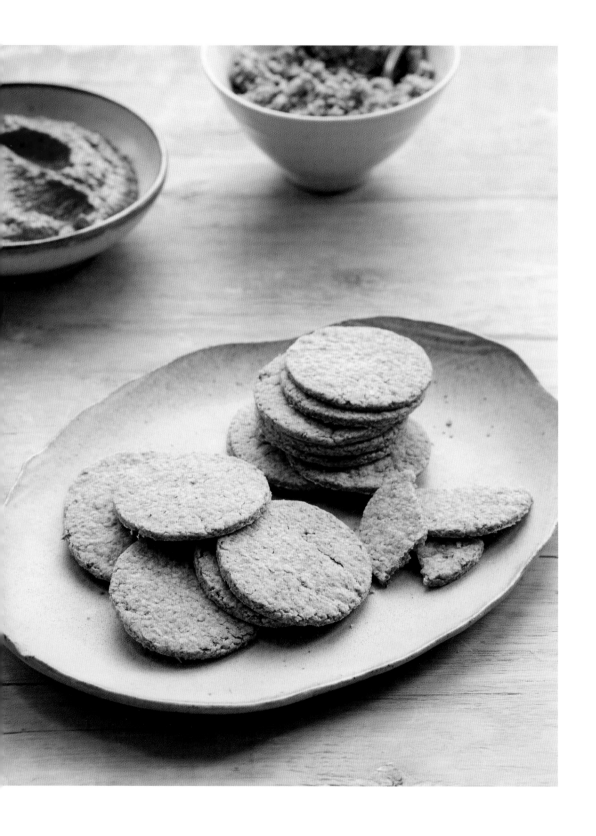

OATCAKES

MAKES 25–35

I love to nibble on something when I'm out and about or on my break at work, and these homemade oatcakes are the perfect snack. They work well teamed with vegetable dips and hummus, cheeses and antipasti, chutney and jams. For bonus points, they're low in sugar but full of fibre and complex carbohydrates, which provide you with a steady stream of energy throughout the day. The quantities below can easily be doubled, so why save one batch of oatcake mixture for a later date?

100g oats

50g wholegrain spelt flour or wholemeal flour, plus extra to dust

¼ tsp salt

1 tsp dried mixed herbs (optional)

2 tbsp light olive oil or rapeseed oil

50–70ml water

Preheat the oven to 180°C/350°F/gas mark 4. Line a baking sheet with baking parchment.

Place the oats in a blender or food processor and blitz for a few seconds, until they resemble a coarse flour. Add the rest of the ingredients, adding the water a bit at a time until the mixture comes together. If the dough feels wet, add a little extra flour.

Lightly flour a work surface and roll out the dough as thinly as you can. Using a 6cm cutter, stamp out small circles (or whatever shapes you fancy). Depending on the thickness and size of your oatcakes, you should be able to make 25–35.

Place on the prepared baking sheet and bake for 20–25 minutes, until lightly golden (be careful they don't burn). Allow to cool completely before storing in an airtight container for 7–10 days.

MINDFUL EATING

When was the last time you sat down to enjoy a meal without any distractions? No phone, laptop, tablet or television; no driving with one hand and lunchbox in the other; no picking from the pot whilst feeding the kids and the dog?

We all have to eat. We are all busy. Most of us eat too much and too quickly; we eat for comfort, from boredom, or simply out of habit because the food is right there. This is normal up to a point because we are only human, but when it's happening daily, in some cases at every meal, we end up feeling too full, or unsatisfied by what we've eaten, not digesting or absorbing our food, and making poor food choices.

Eating has become an automatic behaviour: pick up fork – stab vegetable – open mouth – insert food – chew – scroll Instagram – chew some more – swallow – repeat.

Sound familiar?

As humans, we have a limited mental capacity, so the ability to assign routine tasks to lower-level brain involvement in order to free up space for more cognitively demanding tasks is actually a pretty effective and necessary mechanism for us to evolve as a highly functioning species. Switching to autopilot when we eat may be time-efficient, but it's not doing much for our health. We're not really paying attention to how much we are eating, and most of us will eat the entire portion presented to us regardless of the size and, in some cases, regardless of taste. This theory was investigated in an interesting study (2005) by scientists Brian Wansink and Junying Kim, who randomised a group of 158 cinema-goers into two groups. Each group was given a medium or large box of popcorn; one group's was fresh and the other stale (fourteen days old). They found that those who were given fresh popcorn ate 45.3% more when it was given to them in large rather than medium containers, while those who had stale popcorn still ate 33.6% more when eating from a large container rather than a medium one.

This demonstrates how easy it easy to overeat, and I'm sure you can relate to that, particularly during Christmas time when you're full of turkey and mince pies, but you still can't help making your way through the box of chocolates that's been left on the table.

YOUR FIRST INTRODUCTION TO MINDFUL EATING

Mindful eating is a lot easier than it sounds. You don't need to buy a manual or have any formal training; you just need to pay a little more attention to the here and now. In fact, I'm sure you've done this before. Think about how babies first learn to eat: they are so curious about everything they pick up. They play with the food before they eat it, mushing it between their chubby little hands, and crumbling it onto the table (or floor). They hesitantly taste it before deciding whether they like it enough to eat it, pulling faces of disgust at the foods that don't quite make the cut.

Now think back to your own childhood, eating dinner at the table with your family when your mum wouldn't let you play snake on your phone, watch TV, or fight with your brother over whose turn it was to clean up. Although at the time those designated family mealtimes might have seemed like an inconvenience (especially when they clashed with *The Simpsons*), they taught you how to focus your attention on what you were eating and who you were eating with.

Research shows that families who eat together three or more times per week are less likely to be overweight and are more likely to have healthier dietary and eating patterns than those who share fewer meals.

Meals ought to be golden opportunities to take a break from a working day, the ideal excuse to embrace a nourishing pause, but many people see them as a necessary inconvenience.

- Michael Acton Smith, *Calm*

MINDFUL COOKING

I think cooking from scratch is one of the biggest changes you can make to improve your health and your relationship with food. It encourages you to have a greater variety of foods in your diet, to appreciate food in its raw form, to pick and choose what you love or loathe (coriander in my case), to save money (unless you shop in niche healthfood stores or have a diet rich in lobster), and to cut down on calorie-dense, low-nutrient foods.

The business of preparing and cooking food can in itself be very therapeutic, albeit occasionally stressful. Yes, the process takes time: you have to plan meals, write a list, do the shopping, then set aside time to cook and clean up afterwards. But it also forces you to engage with the recipe from beginning to end, and you soon begin to discover new flavours and textures. You learn how to improvise and rustle up meals from the remnants of your fridge at the end of the week. You experiment and add your own twist to classic recipes or those passed to you by family and friends. Also, setting aside half an hour in the kitchen during the day gives you the opportunity to be mindful.

When I'm being truly present in the kitchen, there's no thinking; my hands and mind are seemingly in perfect concert with one another. You don't get that kind of take-away from a take-away pizza.

MINDFUL EATING EXERCISE

- Take an orange. Examine how it looks, the colour, the texture, the shape.

- Unpeel the orange slowly. How does it feel? Does the skin come away easily, or can you feel resistance from the stringy white membrane?

- Examine the flesh – the shape, texture, colour and any indentations you might have made in the flesh whilst peeling it.

- Now smell the orange and really get a sense of it and its aroma; is the smell strong?

- Separate the segments. Examine their inner structure – hundreds of tiny, juice-filled sacs. How does a segment feel between your fingertips? Is it soft or hard, cold or warm?

- Now close your eyes and place a segment in your mouth without chewing. How does it feel? How does it taste? Finally, bite into it and pay close attention to the explosion of taste in your mouth. Chew slowly and mindfully.

- Eat each segment mindfully and pretend this is the last orange on earth.

NOW ASK YOURSELF:

- Was the orange satisfying? Why or why not?

- What would happen if you ate food this way more often?

- How often do you eat because you are genuinely hungry? How often do you eat to fill a need that has nothing to do with food?

NANNY'S IRISH APPLE TART

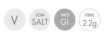

MAKES 8–10 SLICES

The first recipe my mum (pictured with me here) taught me to make was an apple tart, and she first learnt it from her mother. It has been handed down from generation to generation by most families in Ireland. Rarely did we weigh the ingredients because we made it so often when growing up that we quickly learnt how to judge quantities by eye. I even won a prize for it when I was five or six. I hadn't made it in a couple of years until testing it for this book, but my hands quickly remembered what to do. I recently came across Nanny's handwritten notepad, which has all her favourite recipes scribbled down: 'Can make tarts out of anything; apples, rhubarb, gooseberries, B currants, R currants etc. Flour, margarine, sugar, pinch of salt, water + milk.'

225g plain flour, plus extra to dust

125g chilled butter, diced or grated, plus extra to grease

2–3 tbsp cold water, plus extra if necessary

4 large cooking apples, peeled, cored and sliced

Juice of 1 lemon

2 tbsp caster sugar

1 tbsp cornflour

1 tsp ground cinnamon

1 free-range egg, beaten with a splash of milk

Sift the flour into a bowl. Add the butter and rub it in using your fingertips. When the mixture resembles breadcrumbs, pour in the water a bit at a time, mixing until a soft dough forms (you might not need it all). Turn the dough onto a floured board and knead lightly until smooth. Wrap it in cling film and place in the fridge for at least 1 hour.

Meanwhile, peel, core and slice the apples. Place them in a large bowl, add the lemon juice, caster sugar, cornflour and cinnamon and toss well. If you prefer a very soft apple filling, you can put the fruit in a pan with a dash of water and cook it for 3–5 minutes.

Preheat the oven to 190°C/375°F/gas mark 5. Grease a 20cm round ovenproof dish with butter.

Lightly dust a work surface with flour and roll out half the pastry to the size of the prepared dish. Use it to line the plate, letting the excess pastry overhang the edge. Place the apples on it.

Roll out the remaining pastry and use to cover the apples. Using the back of a knife, trim off the excess pastry. Seal the pie by pressing around the edge with a fork.

Reroll the pastry bits to cut out decorative shapes (leaves, stars or whatever) and stick them to the top of the pie with the egg wash. Brush the whole surface with egg wash, then prick 3 or 4 holes in the pastry for steam to escape. Bake for 30–35 minutes, until golden.

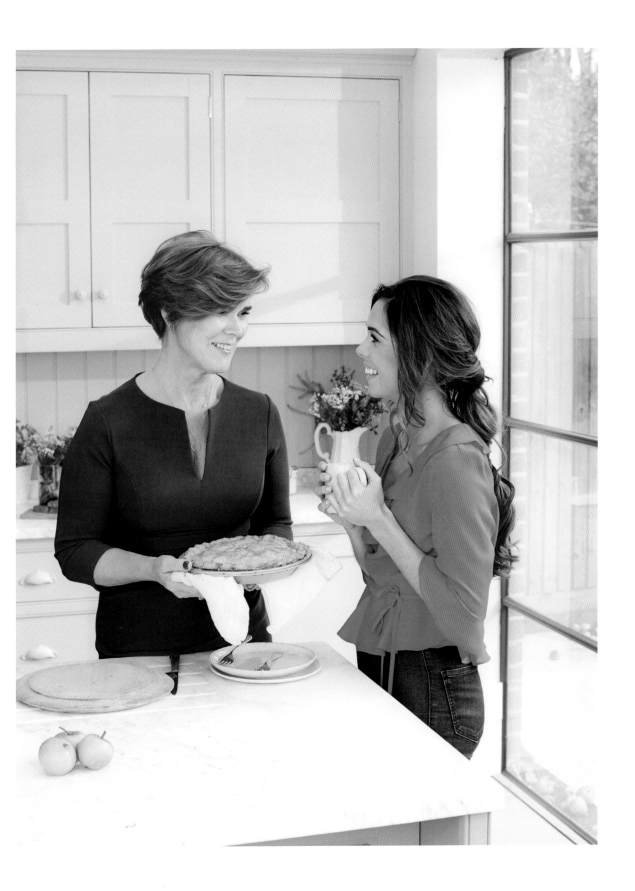

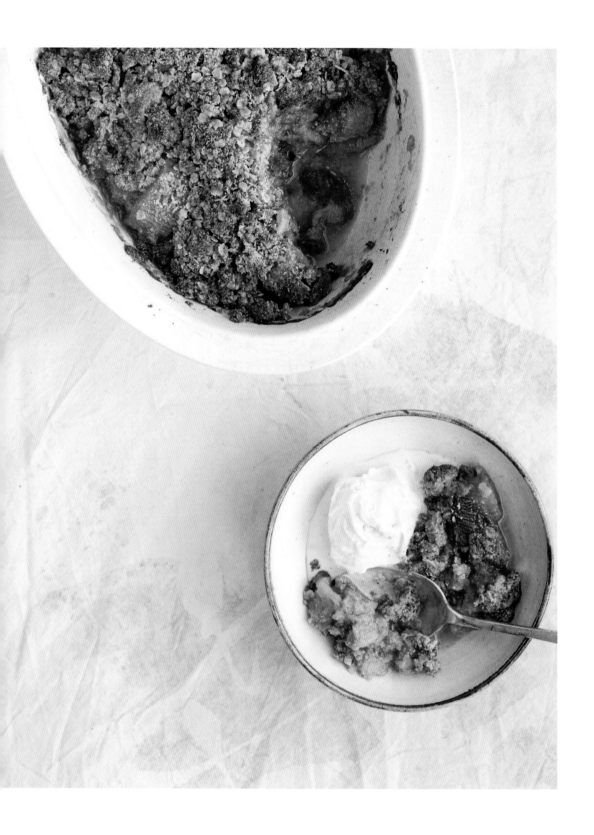

RHUBARB CRUMBLE

SERVES 6

Not everyone likes the sharp flavour of rhubarb, but I love it, especially in this crumble. Rhubarb is also a great source of fibre and important vitamins, such as C and K. Traditionally, my family would serve this crumble with custard and ice cream, but it also tastes incredible with smooth Greek yogurt.

400g rhubarb, trimmed and cut into 3cm chunks

Juice from 1 orange

1 tsp vanilla extract

2 tbsp maple syrup or honey

FOR THE TOPPING

100g ground almonds

50g oats

2 tbsp coconut sugar or brown sugar

1 tsp ground cinnamon

1 tsp ground nutmeg

80g butter or coconut oil, at room temperature

Preheat the oven to 180°C/350°F/gas mark 4. Set out a deep pie dish.

Put the rhubarb in a saucepan with the orange juice, vanilla and maple syrup and cook over a medium heat, until soft but still retaining some shape. Transfer to the pie dish.

Combine the almonds, oats, sugar, cinnamon and nutmeg in a bowl. Add the butter and rub it in with your fingertips until the mixture resembles crumbs. Sprinkle it over the rhubarb.

Bake for 20–25 minutes, until golden. Serve warm with yogurt.

BROWN RICE PUDDING WITH PLUM COMPOTE

SERVES 3–4

'Ooh arr, it's Ambrosia!' Please tell me someone remembers that TV advert with the farmer sitting on a cow singing about his rice pudding? If not, I must sound like a lunatic. I used to have a bowl of rice pudding and a spoon of jam after soccer training when I was younger. In hindsight, it was a really good snack to have after running around because it has carbohydrates from the rice, and protein and calcium from the milk – perfect for growing kids.

225g uncooked brown rice

1 x 400ml tin of reduced-fat coconut milk, or use full-fat if you prefer

2 tsp vanilla extract

1 tsp ground cinnamon

½ tsp ground nutmeg

2 tbsp brown sugar

FOR THE COMPOTE

6 ripe plums, stoned and quartered

1 tbsp brown sugar

2 tbsp water

Cook the rice in a saucepan as per the packet instructions (usually 25 minutes). Drain off any excess water.

Add the coconut milk to the rice, along with the vanilla, spices and sugar. Bring to the boil over a medium heat, then simmer for 8–10 minutes, stirring frequently, until most of the liquid has been absorbed.

To make the compote, place the plums in a small saucepan with the sugar and water. Cook gently, stirring to dissolve the sugar. Cover and simmer for 5–10 minutes, stirring occasionally, until the plums are soft but not mushy. (Plums vary in juiciness, so you can add a splash more water if needed.)

Allow the compote to cool slightly before serving it spooned over the hot rice. Alternatively, let both cool completely, then chill for a couple of hours and eat cold.

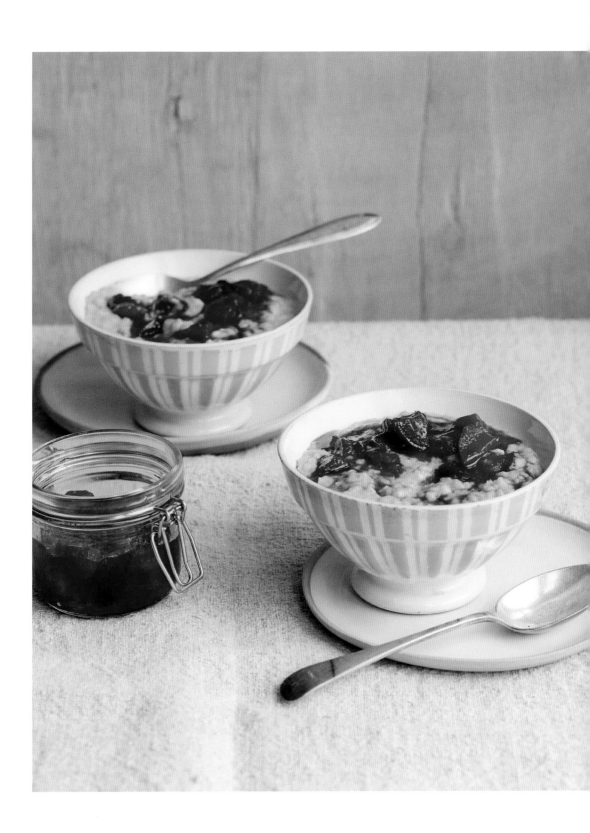

CHOCOLATE + COFFEE MOUSSE ON CRUSHED OATCAKES

SERVES 6

Things I would take to a desert island: coffee and chocolate. The oatcakes add a touch of sophistication.

160g dark chocolate,
  broken into pieces

2 tbsp unsalted butter
  or coconut oil

1 tsp cocoa powder, plus
  extra to dust

30ml cold espresso coffee

8 free-range egg whites,
  at room temperature

Salt

FOR THE BASE

150g Oatcakes
  (see page 215)

4 medjool dates, pitted

4 tbsp coconut oil, melted

Salt

First make the base. Put the oatcakes, dates and a large pinch of salt into a blender or food processor and pulse until finely chopped. Stir through the coconut oil until the mixture resembles wet sand. Divide equally between 6 serving glasses, pressing it into the bottom. Place in the fridge to set.

To make the mousse, place the chocolate and butter in a heatproof bowl set over a saucepan of simmering water and allow to melt. Once melted, stir in the cocoa powder, a pinch of salt and the espresso.

Put the egg whites into a bowl and whisk to form soft peaks. Once the chocolate has cooled a little, fold in a few tablespoons of the egg white until well combined. Gently but thoroughly fold in the rest.

Divide the mixture evenly between the serving glasses and leave to set in the fridge for at least 2 hours.

When ready, dust with extra cocoa powder and serve immediately.

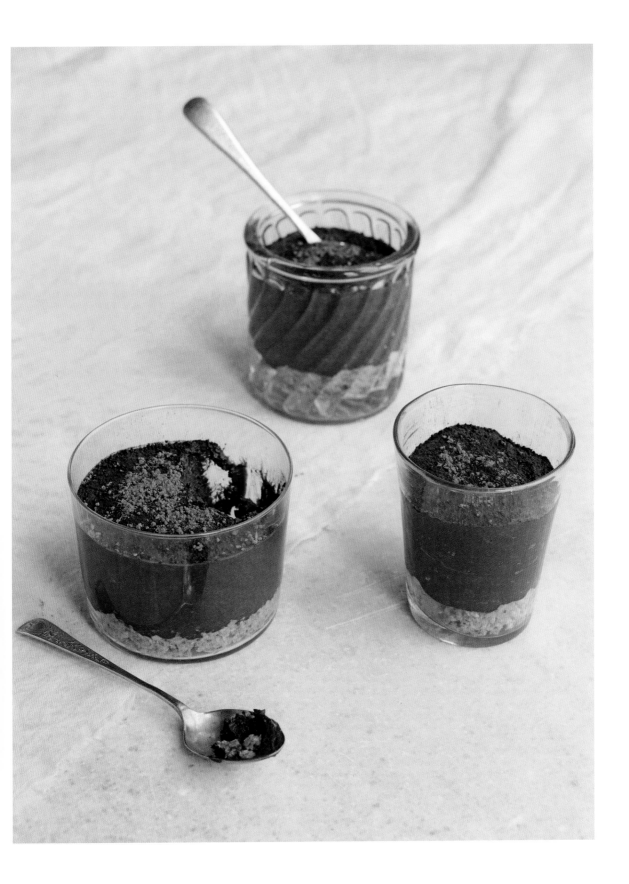

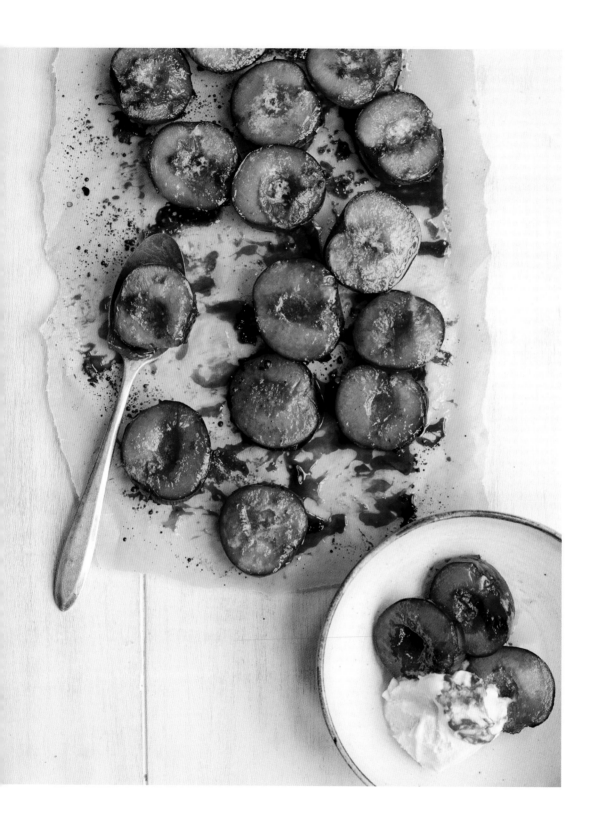

BAKED CINNAMON PLUMS

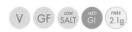

SERVES 4

The smell of butter and cinnamon fills the kitchen when I make this recipe. I'm drooling just thinking about it. This is a really simple crowd-pleaser, but sometimes I just make it for myself if I fancy a quick dessert during the week.

8 plums

1–2 tbsp butter or
    coconut oil

2 tbsp coconut sugar
    or brown sugar

½ tsp ground cinnamon

Natural Greek yogurt,
    coconut yogurt or vanilla
    ice cream, to serve

Preheat the oven to 180°C/350°F/gas mark 4.

Slice the plums in half and remove the stones. Place in an ovenproof dish, flat-side up, and put about a teaspoonful of butter into the middle of each one. Sprinkle the plums with cinnamon and sugar.

Bake for 8–12 minutes, until golden. Serve warm with yogurt or ice cream.

LIME + MINT SORBET

SERVES 6

Here is the perfect summer dinner party dessert. It feels very grown up, especially served in beautiful glasses with mint leaves scattered on top.

500ml water

180g caster sugar

15g mint leaves, plus
   extra to serve

3 limes

Put the water, sugar and 10g of the mint leaves into a pan, bring to the boil, then simmer for 5 minutes. Strain the liquid through a sieve into a bowl, pressing the mint to extract all its moisture, then discard the leaves.

Zest 2 of the limes, add to the bowl, then set aside to cool completely.

Once cool, add the juice of the 3 limes. Finely chop the remaining 5g of mint and add to the bowl. Place in the fridge until well chilled.

Churn your sorbet in an ice-cream maker if you have one. If not, pour the sorbet mixture into a tray and place in the freezer for about 40 minutes, until the edges are beginning to freeze. At this point, use a fork to whisk the edges into the mixture. Repeat this process two or three more times at 40-minute intervals, then allow the sorbet to freeze completely.

For ease of spooning, let the sorbet sit at room temperature for about 10 minutes. Serve in glasses with some extra mint leaves sprinkled on top.

TEATIME TREATS

In Ireland, teatime means cake time! When my siblings and I were growing up and relatives or friends visited our house, my mum would order us to get out the good china. I loved drinking from a delicate teacup, and on the days when I was feeling slightly under the weather, I remember my dad bringing me cups of tea in Mum's good china to help put a smile on my face.

My favourite teatime treats are fluffy Scones (see page 240) piled high with jam and cream, and gorgeous Lemon + Poppyseed Cupcakes (see page 236) – served with a cup of tea, of course!

ALMOND + LEMON CELEBRATION CAKE

MAKES 10–12 SLICES

This is the cake for birthdays, Mother's Day, Sunday dessert, your best friend's baby shower, or just because.

200g unsalted butter, plus extra to grease

225g golden caster sugar

4 free-range eggs, beaten

100ml cow's milk or almond milk

Zest of 2 lemons

150g white spelt flour

150g ground almonds

1½ tsp baking powder

1 tsp bicarbonate of soda

¼ tsp salt

FOR THE ICING

4 tbsp set honey

500g cream cheese

Zest of 2 lemons

2 tbsp coconut oil or unsalted butter, melted

FOR DECORATION

Flaked almonds

Candied citrus peel (optional)

Preheat the oven to 200°C/400°F/gas mark 6. Grease two 18cm springform cake tins and line them with baking parchment.

First make the icing. Place the honey and 125g of the cream cheese in a bowl and beat until combined. Lightly mix in the remainder of the cream cheese, the lemon zest and coconut oil until barely combined (overbeating will make it runny). Cover with cling film and place in the fridge.

To make the cake, place the butter and sugar in a large bowl and beat until light and fluffy. Gradually beat in the eggs, milk and lemon zest, then fold in the remaining ingredients. Divide the mixture equally between the prepared tins.

Bake for 20–25 minutes, until a skewer inserted into the centre of the cakes comes out clean or has no more than one or two small crumbs attached, as it will continue to cook in the tin.

Set aside to cool for 10 minutes, then carefully turn the cakes onto a wire rack to cool completely.

Once the cakes are completely cool, spread half the icing on one of them. Top with the second cake and spread the remaining icing on the surface.

Sprinkle with the flaked almonds and candied citrus peel (if using).

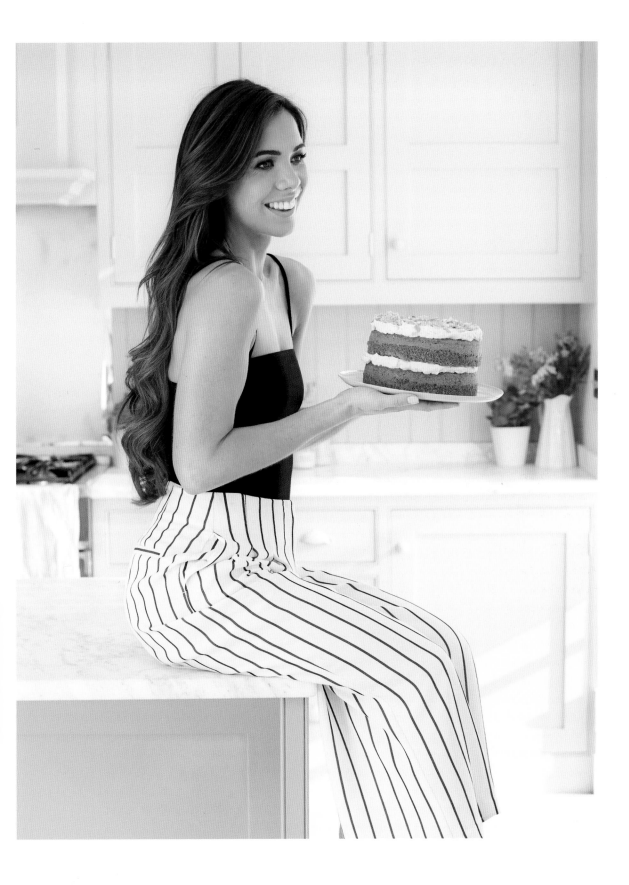

UPSIDE-DOWN SPICED PEAR CAKE

One of my signature dishes has long been an upside-down apple and cinnamon cake, so much so that my family still ask me to make it for them. This is a reinvented version made with pears and spelt flour. It's much nuttier and less sweet than my original recipe, and I hope my family will agree it's even better.

180g unsalted butter,
  plus extra to grease

165g golden caster sugar
  or brown sugar

3 free-range eggs

200ml cow's milk or
  almond milk

280g white spelt flour

100g ground almonds

2 tsp baking powder

½ tsp ground mixed spice

½ tsp ground cinnamon

1 tsp vanilla extract

¼ tsp salt

Natural yogurt, to serve

FOR THE BASE

25g brown sugar

25g butter

½ tsp ground mixed spice

3 ripe pears, peeled, cored
  and halved lengthways

Preheat the oven to 200°C/400°F/gas mark 6. Grease a 23cm springform cake tin and line it with baking parchment.

First make the base. Place the sugar, butter and mixed spice in a bowl and beat together until soft. Spread the mixture in the bottom of the prepared tin, then evenly arrange the pear halves on it, flat-side down. Set aside.

Put the butter and sugar into a bowl and whisk at a high speed until light and fluffy. Beat in the eggs one at a time, and then the milk. Fold in the remaining ingredients and mix thoroughly.

Gently spoon the batter into the cake tin, taking care not to disturb the pears. Smooth the surface, then bake for 35–40 minutes, or until a skewer inserted in the centre comes out clean. Cover with tinfoil if it is browning too quickly.

Set aside to cool in the tin for no longer than 5 minutes, otherwise the pears and sugar will stick to the tin. Invert the cake onto a plate and carefully remove the tin and the baking parchment. Leave to cool completely and serve with yogurt.

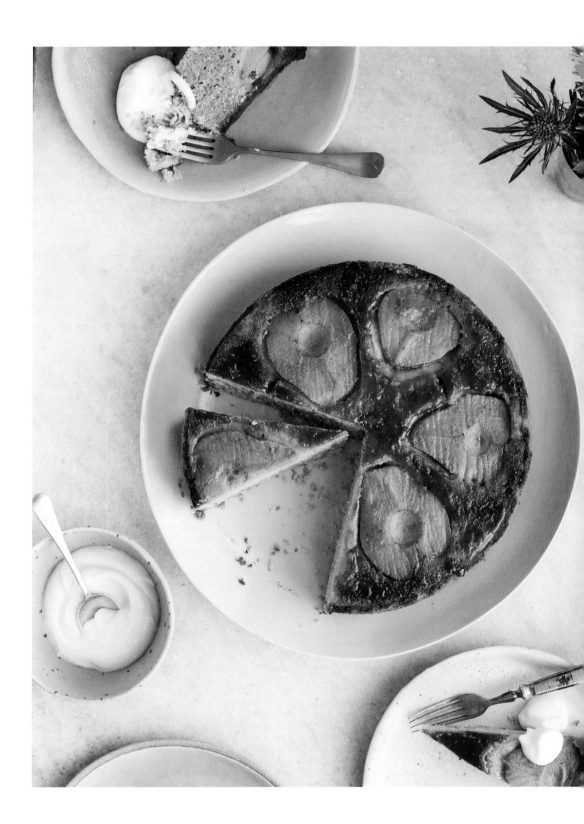

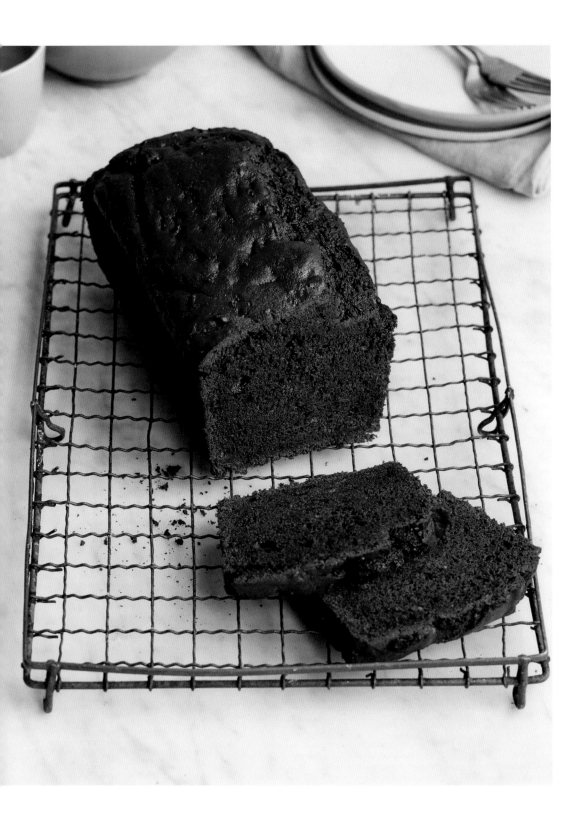

CHOCOLATE + BEETROOT LOAF CAKE

**MAKES A
900G LOAF
(10 SLICES)**

I promise I don't add vegetables to every cake I make, and anyway, adding a vegetable doesn't suddenly make it virtuous. Neither does using natural sugars, such as dates, rather than white sugar. However, this cake may actually offer you some health benefits thanks to the addition of beetroot. Various trials have demonstrated that a compound called dietary nitrate found in beetroot can relax arteries, allowing them to widen and let blood flow with less resistance, thus reducing blood pressure.* We aren't prescribing beetroot juice on the NHS just yet, but watch this space!

100g unsalted butter, at room temperature, plus extra to grease

160g brown sugar

2 free-range eggs, beaten

200g cooked beetroot (see tip, page 84), peeled and coarsely grated

60ml cow's milk or almond milk

200g white spelt flour

1 tsp baking powder

1 tsp bicarbonate of soda

5 tbsp unsweetened cocoa powder

½ tsp salt

1 tsp vanilla extract

50g dark chocolate, melted, to drizzle

Preheat the oven to 200°C/400°F/gas mark 6. Grease a 900g loaf tin and line with baking parchment.

Put the butter and sugar into a large bowl and cream together until light and fluffy. Gradually beat in the eggs, beetroot and milk until well mixed.

Combine all the remaining ingredients (apart from the chocolate) in a separate bowl. Gradually add them to the beetroot mixture, stirring just until they have come together.

Transfer the mixture to the prepared tin and bake for 40–45 minutes, until a skewer inserted in the centre comes out clean. If the top is browning too quickly, cover it with tinfoil.

Set aside to cool in the tin for 10 minutes, then turn onto a wire rack to cool completely.

Drizzle the melted chocolate over the cake and serve immediately.

* Kapil, V., Khambata, R.S., Robertson, A. et al. (2015). Dietary nitrate provides sustained blood pressure lowering in hypertensive patients: a randomized, phase 2, double-blind, placebo-controlled study. Hypertension, vol.65, pp. 320–327.

LEMON + POPPYSEED CUPCAKES

MAKES 12

When I first got into baking, I was very young and would spend hours creating a mess in the kitchen as I made cupcakes, scones and cakes for teatime on a Sunday. Some of you may be wondering why I'm including recipes with ingredients that many would consider 'unhealthy'. Well, no food eaten in moderation is unhealthy. The reason I have used refined sugar rather than honey or a liquid sweetener is because I want fluffy cupcakes, not something dense.

125g unsalted butter or coconut oil, softened

125g golden caster sugar

2 free-range eggs

1 tsp vanilla extract

150g white spelt flour

30g poppy seeds, plus extra to decorate

2 tsp baking powder

Zest of 2 lemons

FOR THE ICING

150g cream cheese

Zest of 2 lemons

50g butter, melted

Preheat the oven to 180°C/350°F/gas mark 4. Line a 12-hole cupcake tray with paper cases.

To make the icing, place all the ingredients in a bowl and beat until combined. Cover with cling film and place in the fridge.

Put the butter and sugar into a bowl and beat at a high speed until light and creamy. Beat in the eggs and vanilla, then slowly beat in the flour, poppy seeds, baking powder and lemon zest.

Divide the mixture equally between the paper cases and bake for 18–20 minutes, until golden and firm to the touch. Set aside and leave to cool.

Just before teatime, spoon or pipe the icing onto the cupcakes. Sprinkle with some poppy seeds, then serve on an attractive plate.

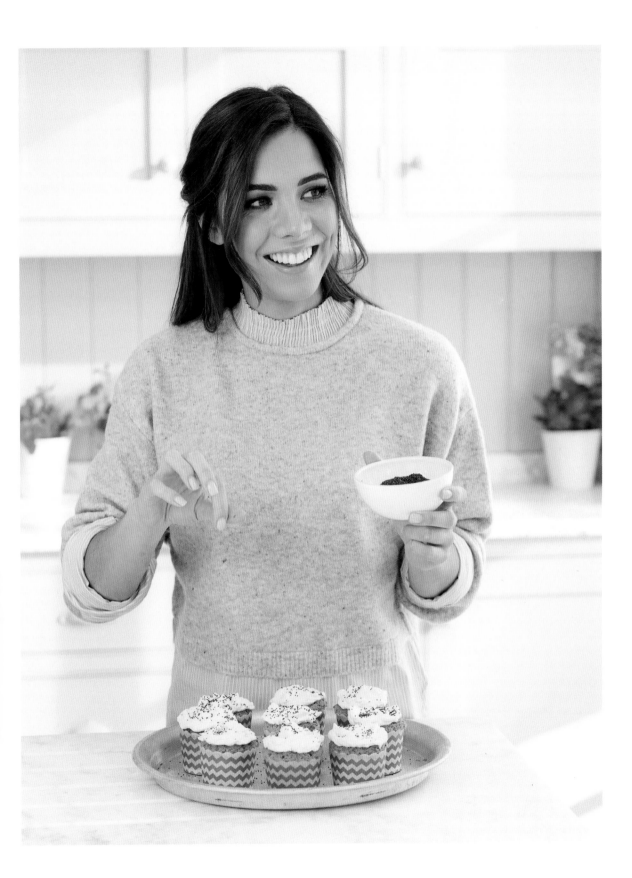

SLEEP

Sleep is non-negotiable. It is just as important to the human body as eating, drinking and breathing. Yet for most of us, it tends to get sidelined. We see it as an indulgence, a luxury that we don't have time for because we could be doing something productive – like watching one more episode on Netflix?

I will be the first to say my sleep habits are far from perfect, and in my late teens I suffered from a very disordered sleeping pattern. You might be thinking, 'That's true of most teenagers, isn't it? They stay up late and sleep in late.' Well, that might not be ideal, but it is not a disordered sleeping pattern *per se*.

It all began shortly after my father died, and although I thought I was coping well by going to school, keeping my grades up and so on, my grief manifested itself in other ways – through weight loss, anxiety and poor sleep.

The core of my sleep problem was insomnia. I simply couldn't get to sleep, and would lie awake for hours, tossing and turning, eventually nodding off around 4am and waking again at 9am feeling worn out. My mum would often find me sitting up watching TV in the early hours of the morning, wrapped in my duvet in the vain hope that I would fall asleep. I even tried listening to ocean sounds, spa music and sleep hypnosis on YouTube, but nothing worked. I would lie in bed crying with exhaustion, but I could not silence my thoughts. I could not switch off.

Often on the nights when I did fall asleep, I would wake up in my bed with an awareness of where I was, but be unable to move – a condition known as sleep paralysis. Eventually, I would come out of my frozen state and release all the air from my lungs in a scream. It is a terrifying experience for anyone who has ever experienced it, and almost more terrifying for anyone else in the house.

Although my attacks of sleep paralysis slowly disappeared when I went to uni, my sleep pattern didn't improve. Now I knew that I could function on just a few hours' sleep every night, I would often stay up late working, or pull all-nighters to make a deadline or revise for exams. I was always tired, but that became my normality. It felt normal not to have the energy for walking up a flight of stairs. It felt normal to have a low-grade headache always grumbling in the background. It felt normal to find no buzz from the ten or twelve coffees I would drink in a day. It felt normal to see my face with a greyish tinge and bags under my eyes. I was a walking zombie and it felt normal! Well, at least until I changed things.

I didn't intentionally set out to sleep better, but when I started changing my lifestyle – exercising daily, eating well, cutting down on stimulants such as coffee and sugar – my sleep improved. Dealing with my grief and coming to terms with losing my father also allowed me to let go of a lot of the angst inside my head that was keeping me up at night.

I'm so much better now. I can't remember the last sleep paralysis attack I had, and I very rarely have a sleepless night. I have a totally different relationship with my bedroom. It used to be my office/library/TV room/storage space, which partly came about from living in cramped student digs for most of my adult life. However, my bedroom is now just my bedroom and I've taken all the clutter out of it. I don't read in bed, write notes, study, or take any devices into my room. It is technology-free and a work-free zone. I get an average of seven hours' sleep a night, which is less than the eight-hour norm, but the quality of that sleep has honestly never been better. I only ever wake in the night if I need to use the bathroom, but, more often than not, I wake up in the same position in which I fell asleep – like a log!

WHY IS SLEEP IMPORTANT?

Lack of sleep doesn't just leave you feeling tired and irritable the next day, it can also reduce how well you think, react, work, learn and get along with others.

Sleep is essential for your brain to work properly, and while you silently sleep, your brain is actually very active, repairing itself and forming new pathways to help you learn and remember information.

Studies show that a good night's sleep improves learning and memory. Whether you're coming to grips with maths, playing an instrument, speaking a new language or driving a car, sleep enhances your learning and problem-solving skills. You might relate to this if you've gone to sleep after studying for an exam, and then dreamt about the things you read and learnt. That's your brain cementing the information for you to access at a later date. So next time you think about pulling an all-nighter before an exam or big presentation, think about how much better off you will be if you simply sleep and allow your brain to catch up with everything you've been trying to remember.

Sleep is not only important for mental sharpness and learning, it also plays an important role in physical health. Research shows that those who get less than seven hours sleep a night on a regular basis are more likely to be overweight or obese, and are at increased risk of developing diabetes, high blood pressure, heart disease and stroke, depression and reduced immune function.

WHAT'S THE MAGIC NUMBER?

There is no magic number, and the amount of sleep required varies depending on age (kids need more than adults), if we are recovering from sleep debt, or if we're sick. For those over the age of eighteen, the recommended amount of sleep is 7–8 hours, but to quote Dr Adrian Williams, the UK's first professor of sleep medicine, one should sleep 'the amount that allows one to wake refreshed and function normally'.

TIPS FOR GETTING A RESTFUL NIGHT'S SLEEP

- Have a tech curfew one hour before bed. Switching off laptops, phones, TVs and tablets before bed will reduce your exposure to the artificial blue light these devices emit. Blue light suppresses the sleep-inducing hormone melatonin, which tricks the brain and body into thinking it's still daytime and they should therefore still be alert. Powering down devices before bedtime signals the brain to start producing melatonin as we prepare to sleep.

- Avoid alcohol last thing. Although a nightcap before bed might help you to fall asleep more quickly, the quality of sleep is reduced, so you end up feeling less rested the following day.

- Avoid high-intensity exercise before bed. Regular exercise has been shown to improve sleep overall, but a high-intensity workout late in the evening could be keeping you up. Our levels of cortisol, a stress hormone, are highest in the morning around 6am, when we need to get up and go to work. They gradually decrease throughout the day, and are lowest in the evening, so we can chill out and go to sleep. However, putting the body under physical or mental stress late in the evening can disrupt this and keep the cortisol levels high, therefore keeping us alert and ready for action. If you can work out only in the evening, give yourself at least an hour to cool down and unwind before bed.

- Have a sleep routine. Having a routine before bed is another strong signal to your body and mind that it's time to power down for the evening. Download a pre-sleep relaxation meditation or a mindfulness podcast, have a bath, light some candles, do some stretching, write in a journal – make it personal to you and do whatever makes you unwind.

- Turn down the lights. Switching off the main lights in favour of lamps or candles sends a signal to the brain to start producing melatonin. It might sound a bit obvious, but having good-quality blackout blinds or curtains in your bedroom will prevent your sleep being disrupted by neighbourhood lights and early morning sun. When it's time to wake up, take yourself outside to suppress your melatonin levels and boost your feel-good hormone, serotonin.

MIXED BERRY + CINNAMON SCONES

**MAKES 8–10
SCONES**

*Scone pronounced like 'stone' or 'ston'? I go with the former, but we won't
fight over it, especially once you taste my delicious recipe for them. I got
the inspiration for these scones from Avoca, a family-run café and food
market in Ireland. When I fly into Dublin I head straight to their café
at Malahide Castle for a scone with jam and a cup of tea.*

220g white spelt flour,
  plus extra to dust

60g caster sugar

1 tsp ground cinnamon

1 tsp baking powder

1 tsp bicarbonate of soda

60g chilled butter or
  coconut oil, plus extra
  to serve

150g mixture of raspberries
  and blueberries

60ml cow's milk or
  almond milk

1 free-range egg, beaten
  with a splash of milk

Salt

Preheat the oven to 180°C/350°F/gas mark 4. Line a baking sheet with
baking parchment.

Place the flour in a large bowl and add the sugar, cinnamon, baking
powder, bicarbonate of soda and a pinch of salt. Cut the butter into
pieces and rub it into the flour until the mixture resembles breadcrumbs.

Cut the raspberries in half and add to the flour mixture along with the
blueberries. Pour in the milk and mix with a spoon, then use your hands
to gently bring it all together into a ball of dough. Take care not to press it
too firmly, or the berries will release their juices, resulting in a wet dough.

Dust your work surface with a little extra flour and roll or pat the dough
out to a thickness of about 3cm. Use a 5cm cutter, glass or lid to stamp
out 8–10 circles, dipping it in flour as you go to prevent things sticking.
Squeeze the leftover scraps of dough together, then roll or pat out as
before and stamp out more circles.

Place the circles of dough on the prepared baking sheet and brush with
a little egg wash. Bake for 15 minutes, until risen and golden. Transfer
to a rack to cool.

The scones will keep for up to 3 days in an airtight container. Reheat
them in the oven or microwave just before serving.

BLUEBERRY CHIA JAM

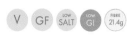

**MAKES 1 X
500G JAR**

Homemade jam is full of nostalgia for me. I remember making blackberry jam with Nanny, my grandmother. My sister and I would pick the berries from the blackberry bushes in the field by our house, using the bottom of our T-shirts as containers (much to Mum's dismay), and carry them back home. Although there is nothing quite like old-fashioned jam, it does contain quite a lot of added sugar, which isn't great for our teeth or health if we eat too much of it. Chia seed jam is a quick, low-sugar alternative – ideal for diabetics – and any frozen fruit will work with this recipe. You can whip it up in just a few minutes and it will keep in the fridge for a couple of weeks.

500g frozen blueberries

2 tbsp water

2 tbsp honey or maple syrup

40g chia seeds

EXTRA FLAVOURINGS (OPTIONAL)

1 tsp ground cinnamon

1 tsp drops vanilla extract

1 tsp ground cardamom

Put the berries and water in a saucepan over a medium heat and cook until the fruit breaks down and becomes syrupy, 5–10 minutes. Mash the fruit with the back of a wooden spoon or a potato masher. I like my jam to have lumps, but you can blend the mixture until smooth if you prefer.

Stir in the honey and chia seeds, and any spices or flavourings you wish to use. Cook for another 2–3 minutes, then remove from heat and leave to stand for 5 minutes, until thickened. If you'd like a thicker consistency, especially with very juicy fruits, stir in more chia seeds a teaspoonful at a time.

Once the jam has cooled to room temperature, transfer it to a sterilised jar (see tip below). Seal tightly, then label and date. The jam will keep in the fridge for 2 weeks, or in the freezer for 3 months.

VARIATION: *Fresh fruit can be used instead of frozen, but it needs slightly longer cooking to release enough juice, and you shouldn't require as many chia seeds.*

TIP: *When potting up jam, it's very important to use sterilised jars (and lids) or the contents can go mouldy. To do this, you can put them through the hottest cycle in a dishwasher. Alternatively, wash them thoroughly in hot water, allow to dry naturally, then place them upside-down in an oven preheated to the lowest possible temperature and leave for about 30 minutes.*

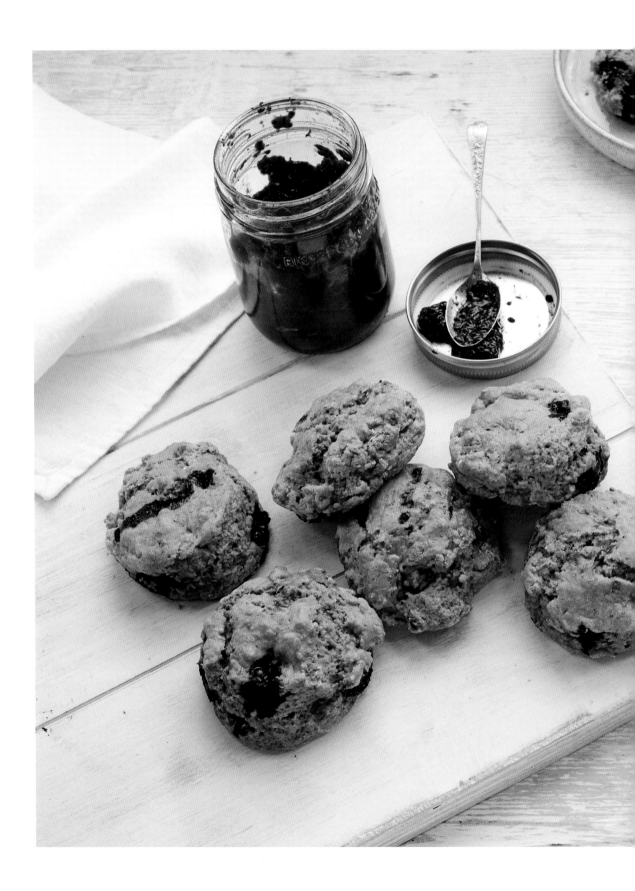

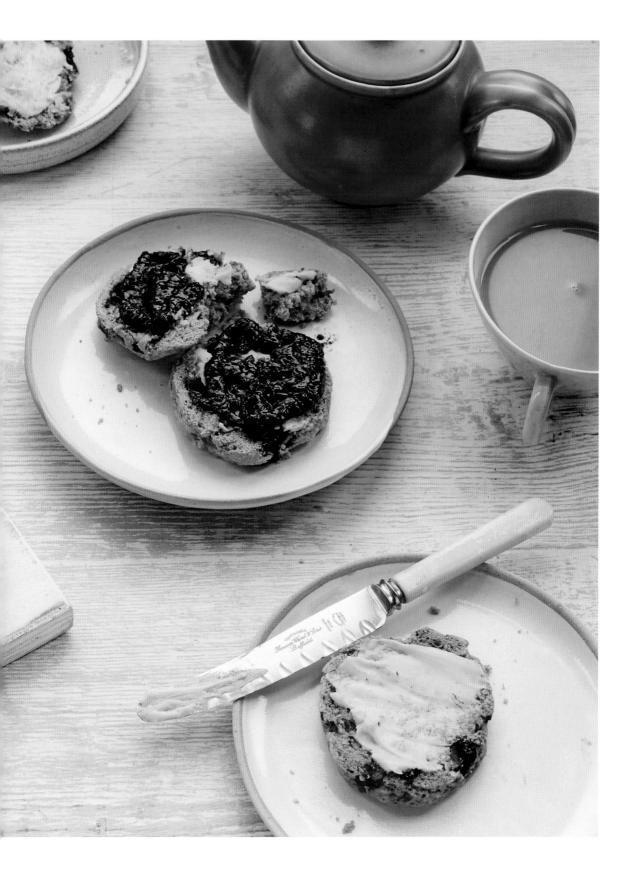

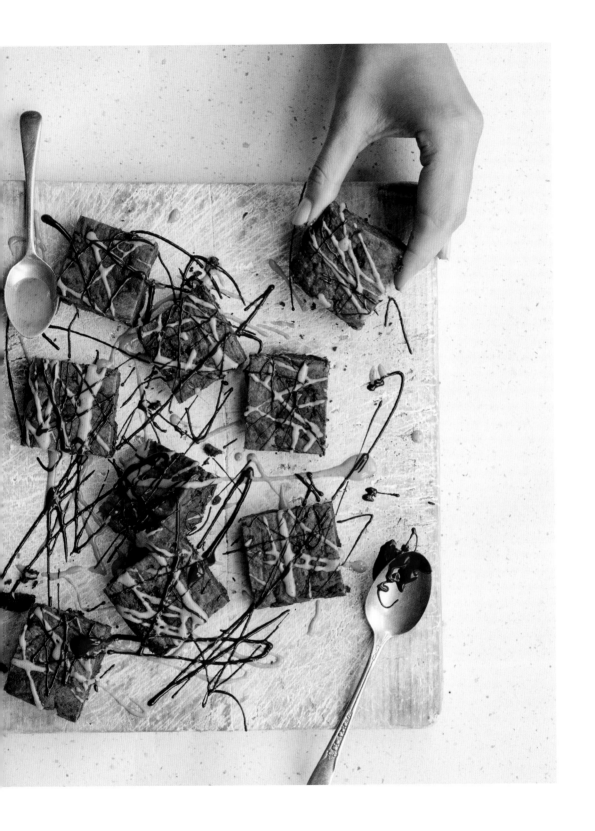

PEANUT BUTTER +
CHICKPEA BLONDIES

MAKES 8–9

Who knew chickpeas could be so versatile? Being high in fibre and protein, they add great texture to these white brownies, and the overall recipe is relatively low in sugar compared to shop-bought versions. I'm not quite sure which tastes better, the raw batter or the cooked blondies, but licking the spoon is definitely one of the best bits of making this recipe.

1 tbsp coconut oil, plus
    extra to grease

1 x 400g tin of chickpeas,
    drained and rinsed

125g smooth peanut butter

4 tbsp milk or water

2 tsp vanilla extract

90ml maple syrup or honey

½ tsp salt

½ tsp baking powder

¼ tsp bicarbonate of soda

60g dark chocolate,
    chopped

1 tbsp cocoa powder

Preheat the oven to 200°C/400°F/gas mark 6. Grease a shallow 15cm square or round baking tin.

Place the chickpeas in a blender or food processor and add the peanut butter, milk, vanilla, maple syrup, salt, baking powder and bicarbonate of soda. Blitz until smooth.

Stir in the chocolate, then tip the batter into the prepared tin.

Melt the tablespoon of coconut oil in a small bowl set over a saucepan of simmering water. Stir in the cocoa powder, then drizzle half the chocolate sauce over the batter and swirl it through the mixture with a knife.

Bake for 16–18 minutes. Set aside to cool in the tin for 15 minutes, then turn onto a wire rack to cool completely.

When ready to serve, cut into squares and drizzle over some more peanut butter and the remaining chocolate sauce. Store in an airtight container in the fridge for up to a week.

CHOCOLATE CHIP BANANA LOAF

**MAKES A
900G LOAF
(10 SLICES)**

As this recipe is less 'cakey' than other banana breads, I call it a loaf. It slices really well, so I like to do this and then freeze it so that I can eat it a slice at a time (simply defrosted or toasted), whenever I feel the need for a treat. It's not awfully sweet, so you can top it with jam or honey. For a lower-sugar version, use chopped nuts instead of chocolate chips.

Butter or coconut oil,
  to grease
230g wholegrain spelt flour
70g oats
1 tsp baking powder
2 tsp ground cinnamon
2 free-range eggs
70g honey or maple syrup
1 tbsp olive oil
100g peanut butter or
  almond butter
2 bananas, mashed
120ml milk
80g chocolate chips

Preheat the oven to 200°C/400°F/gas mark 6. Grease a 900g loaf tin and line it with baking parchment.

Place the flour, oats, baking powder and cinnamon in a bowl and combine.

Beat the eggs in a separate bowl. Add the honey, oil, peanut butter, bananas and milk and beat again. Pour into the flour mixture and stir together. Mix in the chocolate chips.

Pour the mixture into the prepared tin and bake for 45 minutes, until golden on the top and a skewer inserted in the centre comes out clean. (Cover with tinfoil if it is browning too quickly on top.) Transfer to a wire rack to cool.

This bread with keep for up to 3 days in an airtight plastic container, or can be frozen for up to 3 months.

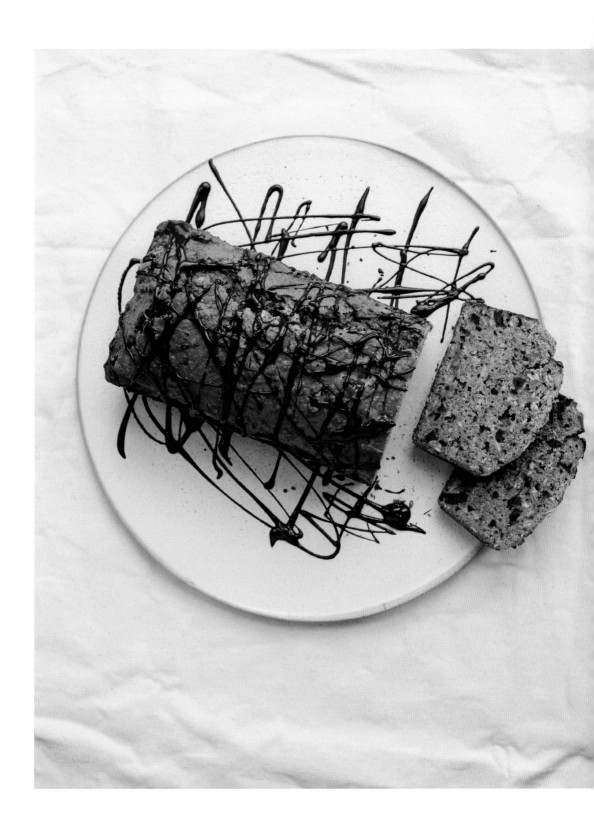

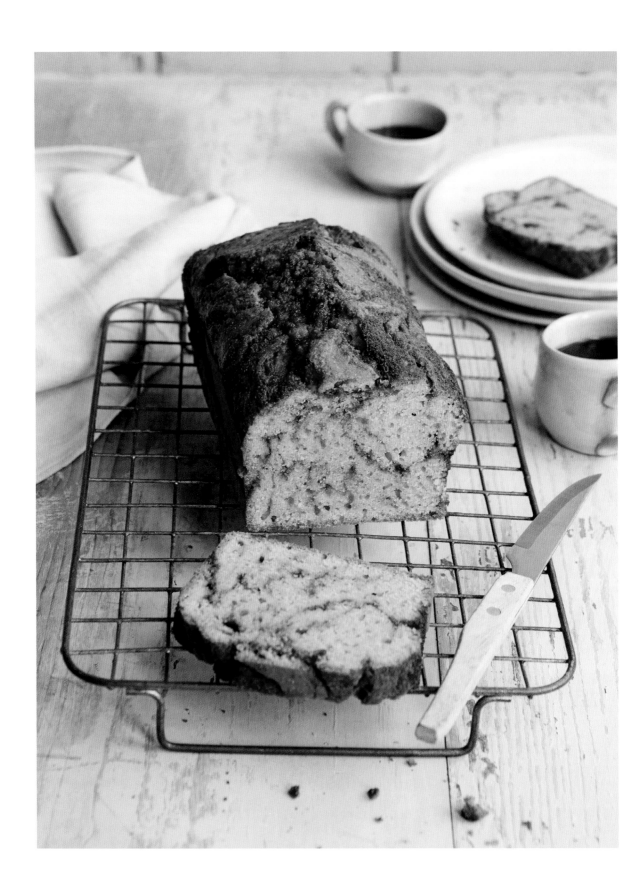

CINNAMON SWIRL LOAF

**MAKES A
900G LOAF
(10 SLICES)**

If you've been to New York, you will know about the cinnamon swirls you can get there. They are massive and smothered in sweet white frosting. They taste great, but I'm pretty sure you get a week's worth of calories and sugar in one bite. This loaf is reminiscent of American cinnamon swirls, but less over the top.

100g unsalted butter or
   coconut oil, melted,
   plus extra to grease
250g white spelt flour
100g ground almonds
200g brown sugar
2 tsp baking powder
¼ tsp salt
3 free-range eggs
160ml cashew or
   almond milk
2 tsp ground cinnamon
Natural yogurt, to serve

Preheat the oven to 180°C/350°F/gas mark 4. Grease a 900g loaf tin and line it with baking parchment.

Place the flour in a large bowl and add the ground almonds, 150g of the sugar, the baking powder and salt. Stir to combine.

Put the eggs, milk and butter in a separate bowl and beat together. Add to the dry mixture and fold together until thoroughly combined.

Pour half the batter into the prepared loaf tin. Smooth it out, then sprinkle with half the remaining sugar and half the cinnamon. Pour the remaining batter on top and sprinkle with the remaining sugar and cinnamon.

Dip a butter knife into the tin and swirl it around a few times to distribute the layers of sugar and cinnamon through the mixture, then smooth the surface.

Bake for 50–55 minutes, until golden brown and a skewer inserted in the centre comes out clean. Cover with tinfoil if it is browning too quickly.

Set aside to cool in the tin for 10 minutes, then turn onto a wire rack to cool completely.

Serve in thick slices with yogurt.

REFERENCES

INTRODUCTION

- Allen, J.C., Corbitt, A.D., Maloney, K.P., Butt, M.S., Truong, V-D. (2012). Glycemic Index of Sweet Potato as Affected by Cooking Methods. *The Open Nutrition Journal*, vol. 6, pp. 1–11.
- Atkinson, F.S., Foster-Powell, K., Brand-Miller, J.C. (2008). International Tables of Glycemic Index and Glycemic Load Values: 2008. *Diabetes Care*, vol. 31(12), pp. 2281–2283.
- Berger, S. Raman, G. Vishwanathan, R., Jacques, P.F., Johnson, E.J. (2015). Dietary cholesterol and cardiovascular disease: a systematic review and meta-analysis. *The American Journal of Clinical Nutrition*, vol. 102, pp. 276–294.
- Bhupathiraju, S.N., Tobias, D.K., Malik, V.S., Pan, A., Hruby, A., Manson, J.E., Willett, W.C., Hu, F.B. (2014). Glycemic index, glycemic load, and risk of type 2 diabetes: results from 3 large US cohorts and an updated meta-analysis. *The American Journal of Clinical Nutrition*, vol. 100(1), pp. 218–232.
- Brand-Miller, J. (2017). *The International Glycemic Index (GI) Database.* (The University of Sydney) Available at: http://www.glycemicindex.com/ [Accessed 8 January 2018].
- Brand-Miller, J., Hayne, S., Petocz, P. Colagiuri, S. (2003). Low–Glycemic Index Diets in the Management of Diabetes. *Diabetes Care*, vol. 26(8), pp. 2466–2468.
- Brand-Miller, J. et al. (2003). *The New Glucose Revolution.* (New York: Marlowe & Company).
- British Heart Foundation. Instant or traditional porridge? Available at: https://www.bhf.org.uk/heart-matters-magazine/nutrition/ask-the-expert/porridge [Accessed 8 January 2018].
- Davis, C., Bryan, J., Hodgson, J., Murphy, K. (2015). Definition of the Mediterranean Diet: A Literature Review. *Nutrients*, vol. 7(11), pp. 9139–9153.
- Dernini, S., Berry, E.M. (2015). Mediterranean diet: from a healthy diet to a sustainable dietary pattern. *Frontiers in Nutrition*, vol. 2, p. 15.
- Food Standards Agency, (2005 [updated 2010]). 8 tips for making healthier choices. [PDF] Available at: https://www.food.gov.uk/sites/default/files/multimedia/pdfs/publication/eatwell0708.pdf [Accessed 8 January 2018].
- Heart UK, (2009). Fact Sheet – The Power of Beta Glucan. [PDF] Available at: https://heartuk.org.uk/images/uploads/healthylivingpdfs/HUK_factsheet_F09_OatBetaGlucanF.pdf [Accessed 8 January 2018].
- McNamara, D.J. (2015). The Fifty Year Rehabilitation of the Egg. *Nutrients*, vol. 7(10), pp. 8716–8722.
- Mondazzi, L. Arcelli, E. (2009). Glycemic Index in Sports Performance. *Journal of American College of Nutrition*, vol. 28(4), pp. 455S-463S.
- Othman, R.A., Moghadasian, M.H., Jones, PJ.H. (2014). Cholesterol-lowering effects of oat -glucan. *Nutrition Reviews*, vol. 69(6), pp. 299–309.
- Sacks, F.M., Lichtenstein, A.H., Wu, J.H.Y., Appel, LJ., Creager, M.A., Kris-Etherton, P.M., Miller, M., Rimm, E.B., Rudel, L.L., Robinson, J.G., Stone, N.J., Van Horn, L.V. on behalf of the American Heart Association. (2017). Dietary Fats and Cardiovascular Disease: A Presidential Advisory from the American Heart Association. *Circulation*, vol. 136(3), pp. e1–e23.
- UNESCO. (2013). Mediterranean Diet. Available at: https://ich.unesco.org/en/RL/mediterranean-diet-00884 [Accessed 8 January 2018].
- United States Department of Agriculture, (2016). Basic Report: 16070, Lentils, mature seeds, cooked, boiled, without salt. Available at: https://ndb.nal.usda.gov/ndb/foods/w/4808?fgcd=&manu=&lfacet=&format=&count=&max=50&offset=&sort=default&order=asc&qlookup=16070&ds=&qt=&qp=&qa=&qn=&q=&ing= [Accessed 8 January 2018].
- Wallace, T. C., Murray, R., Zelman, K.M. (2016). The Nutritional Value and Health Benefits of Chickpeas and Hummus. *Nutrients*, vol. 8(12), p. 766.

MACRONUTRIENTS

- Akter, K., Lanza, E.A., Martin, S.A., Myronyuk, N., Rua, M., Raffa, R.B. (2011). Diabetes mellitus and Alzheimer's disease: shared pathology and treatment? *British Journal of Clinical Pharmacology*, vol. 71(3), pp. 365–376.
- Alzheimer's Society. Facts for the media. [Online] Available at https://www.alzheimers.org.uk/info/20027/news_and_media/541/facts_for_the_media [Accessed 8 January 2018].
- BDA. (2017). Food Fact Sheet – Trans Fats. [PDF] Available at: https://www.bda.uk.com/foodfacts/TransFats.pdf [Accessed 8 January 2018].
- Buttriss, J. (2015). Why 5%? [PDF] (London: Public Health England). Available at: https://www.gov.uk/government/uploads/system/uploads/attachment_data/file/489906/Why_5__-_The_Science_Behind_SACN.pdf [Accessed 8 January 2018].
- British Nutrition Foundation. (2012). Protein. [Online] Available at: https://www.nutrition.org.uk/nutritionscience/nutrients-food-and-ingredients/protein.html [Accessed 8 January 2018].
- Bean, A. (2017). The Complete Guide to Sports Nutrition, 8th ed. (London: Bloomsbury Publishing).
- Daviglus, M.L., Bell, C.C., Berrettini, W., Bowen, P.H., Sander Connolly, E., Cox, N.J., Dunbar-Jacob, J.M., Granieri, E.C., Hunt, G., McGarry, K., Patel, D., Potosky, A.L., Sanders-Bush, E., Silberburg, D., Trevisan, M. (2010). National Institutes of Health State-of-the-Science Conference Statement: Preventing Alzheimer Disease and Cognitive Decline. *Annals of Internal Medicine*, vol. 153, pp. 176–181.
- de la Monte, S.M., Wands, J.R. (2008). Alzheimer's Disease Is Type 3 Diabetes – Evidence Reviewed. *Journal of Diabetes Science and Technology*, vol. 2(6), pp. 1101–1113.
- de Souza, R.J., Mente, A., Maroleanu, A., Cozma, A.L., Ha, V., Kishibe, T., Uleryk, E., Budylowski, P., Schünemann, H., Beyene, J., Anand, S.S. (2015). Intake of saturated and trans unsaturated fatty acids and risk of all cause mortality, cardiovascular disease, and type 2 diabetes: systemic review and meta-analysis of observational studies. *BMJ*, vol. 351, p. h3978.
- Diabetes UK. What is Type 1 diabetes? [Online] Available at: https://www.diabetes.org.uk/diabetes-the-basics/what-is-type-1-diabetes [Accessed 8 January 2018].
- Diabetes UK. (2016). New diabetes prevalence figures for England. [Online] Available at: https://www.diabetes.org.uk/about_us/news/new-diabetes-prevalence-figures-for-england [Accessed 8 January 2018].

- Lincoln, P. (2010). NICE PDG: The prevention of cardiovascular disease at a population level. [PDF] *NICE*. Available at: https://www.nice.org.uk/guidance/ph25/evidence/expert-paper-9-trans-fats-pdf-373069117 [Accessed 8 January 2018].
- Laaninen, T. (2016). Trans Fats – Overview of recent developments. *EPRS* [PDF] Available at: http://www.europarl.europa.eu/RegData/etudes/BRIE/2016/577966/EPRS_BRI(2016)577966_EN.pdf [Accessed 8 January 2018].
- López-Miranda, J., Badimon, L., Bonanome, A., Lairon, D., Kris-Etherton, P.M., Mata, P., Pérez-Jiménez, F. (2014). Monounsaturated Fat and Cardiovascular Risk. *Nutrition Reviews*, vol. 64(4), pp. s2–s12.
- Mozaffarian D., Katan M.B., Ascherio, A., Stampfer, M.J., Willett W.C. (2006). Trans fatty acids and cardiovascular disease. *New England Journal of Medicine*, vol. 354, pp. 1601–1613.
- Ravona-Springer, R., Schnaider-Beeri, M. (2011). The association of diabetes and dementia and possible implications for nondiabetic populations. *HHS Public Access*, vol. 11(11), pp. 1609–1617.
- Sacks, F.M., Lichtenstein, A.H., Wu, J.H.Y., Appel, L.J., Creager, M.A., Kris-Etherton, P.M., Miller, M., Rimm, E.B., Rudel, L.L., Robinson, J.G., Stone, N.J., Van Horn, L.V. on behalf of the American Heart Association. (2017). Dietary Fats and Cardiovascular Disease: A Presidential Advisory From the American Heart Association. *Circulation*, vol. 137(2), pp. e1–e23.
- SACN. (2007). Update on trans fatty acids and health. TSO [PDF] Available at: https://www.gov.uk/government/uploads/system/uploads/attachment_data/file/339359/SACN_Update_on_Trans_Fatty_Acids_2007.pdf [Accessed 8 January 2018].
- SACN. (2015). SACN Carbohydrates and Health Report. [Online] Available at: https://www.gov.uk/government/publications/sacn-carbohydrates-and-health-report [Accessed 8 January 2018].
- Samaras, K., Sachdev, P.S. (2012). Diabetes and the elderly brain: sweet memories? *Therapeutic Advances in Endocrinology and Metabolism*, vol. 3(6), pp. 189–196.
- Threapleton, D.E., Greenwood, D.C., Evans, C.E.L., Cleghorn, C.L., Nykjaer, C., Woodhead, C., Cade, J.E., Gale, C.P., Burley, V.J. (2013). Dietary fibre intake and risk of cardiovascular disease: systematic review and meta-analysis. *BMJ*, vol. 347, p. f6879.

MICRONUTRIENTS

- Aprotosoaie, A.C., Miron, A., Trifan, A., Luca, V.S., Costache, I-I. (2016). The Cardiovascular Effects of Cocoa Polyphenols – An Overview. *Diseases*, vol. 4(4), p. 39.
- BDA, (2016). Food Fact Sheet – Vitamin D. [PDF] Available at: https://www.bda.uk.com/foodfacts/VitaminD.pdf [Accessed 8 January 2018].
- BDA, (2017). Food Fact Sheet – Calcium. [PDF] Available at: https://www.bda.uk.com/foodfacts/Calcium.pdf [Accessed 8 January 2018].
- Habauzit, V., Monrand, C. (2012). Evidence for a protective effect of polyphenols-containing food on cardiovascular health: an update for clinicians. *Therapeutic Advances in Chronic Disease*, vol. 3(2), pp. 87–106.
- Johnson, E.J. (2002). The role of carotenoids in human health. *Nutrition in clinical care*, vol. 5(2), pp. 56–65.
- Manach, C., Scalbert, A., Morand, C., Rémésy,C., Jiménez, L. (2004). Polyphenols: food sources and bioavailability. *The American Journal of Clinical Nutrition*, vol. 79(5), pp. 727–747.
- Mellor, D.D., Madden, L.A., Smith, K.A., Kilpatrick, E.S. Atkin, S.L. (2013). High-polyphenol chocolate reduces endothelial dysfunction and oxidative stress during acute transient hyperglycaemia in Type 2 diabetes: a pilot randomized controlled trial. *Diabetic Medicine*, vol. 30(4). pp. 478–483.
- Nutrilite Health Institute. Global Phytonutrient Report. 2014. Available at: https://www.amwayglobal.com/wp/wp-content/uploads/2017/09/global_phytonutrient_report_commissioned_by_the_nutrilite_health_institute.pdf [Accessed 8 January 2018].
- Public Health England, (2016). Press release – PHE publishes new advice on vitamin D. Available at: https://www.gov.uk/government/news/phe-publishes-new-advice-on-vitamin-d [Accessed 8 January 2018].
- Ried, K., Fakler, P, Stocks, N.P. (2017). Effect of cocoa on blood pressure. *The Cochrane Database of Systematic Reviews*. [Online] Available at: https://www.ncbi.nlm.nih.gov/pubmed/28439881 [Accessed 8 January 2018].
- Rimbach, G., Melchin, M., Moehring, J., Wagner, A.E. (2009). Polyphenols from Cocoa and Vascular Health – A Critical Review. *International Journal of Molecular Sciences*, vol. 10(10), pp. 4290–4309.
- SACN, (2016). Vitamin D and Health. [PDF] Available at: https://www.gov.uk/government/uploads/system/uploads/attachment_data/file/537616/SACN_Vitamin_D_and_Health_report.pdf [Accessed 8 January 2018].
- Schroeter, H., Heiss, C., Spencer, J.P.E., Keen, C.L., Lupton, J.R., Schmitz, H.H. (2010). Recommending flavanols and procyanidins for cardiovascular health: Current knowledge and future needs. *Molecular Aspects of Medicine*, vol. 31(6), pp. 546–557.
- Vinson, J.A., Motisi, M.J. (2015). Polyphenol antioxidants in commercial chocolate bars: Is the label accurate? *Journal of Functional Foods*, vol. 12, pp. 526–529.

FIBRE + GUT HEALTH

- Food and Agriculture Organization of the United Nations. (2004). What is happening to agrobiodiversity? [Online] Available at: http://www.fao.org/docrep/007/y5609e/y5609e02.htm [Accessed 8 January 2018].

IS FIVE-A-DAY ENOUGH ?

- Aune, D., Giovannucci, E., Boffetta, P., Fadnes, L.T., Keum, N., Norat, T., Greenwood, D.C., Riboli, E., Vatten, L.J., Tonstad, S. (2017). Fruit and vegetable intake and the risk of cardiovascular disease, total cancer and all-cause mortality – a systematic review and dose-response meta-analysis of prospective studies. *International Journal of Epidemiology*, vol. 46(3), pp. 1029–1056.
- British Heart Foundation. Heart Statistics. [Online] Available at: https://www.bhf.org.uk/research/heart-statistics [Accessed 8 January 2018].
- NHS. Food Fact Sheet – Fruit and vegetables – how to get five-a-day. [PDF] Available at: http://www.nhs.uk/Livewell/5ADAY/Documents/Downloads/5ADAY_portion_guide.pdf [Accessed 8 January 2018].
- NHS Choices. (2015). Why 5 a Day? [Online] Available at: http://www.nhs.uk/Livewell/5ADAY/Pages/Why5ADAY.aspx [Accessed 8 January 2018].
- Public Health England. (2016). National Diet and Nutrition Survey – Results from Years 5 and 6 (combined) of the Rolling Programme (2012/2013–2013/2014). [PDF] Available at: https://www.gov.uk/government/uploads/system/uploads/attachment_data/file/551352/NDNS_Y5_6_UK_Main_Text.pdf [Accessed 8 January 2018].

VEGETARIAN + VEGAN DIETS

- Bazzano, L.A., He. J., Ogden, L.G., Loria, C.M., Vupputuri, S., Myers, L., Whelton, P.K. (2002). Fruit and vegetable intake and risk of cardiovascular disease inUS adults: the first National Health and Nutrition Examination Survey Epidemiologic Follow-up Study. *The American Journal of Clinical Nutrition*, vol. 76(1), pp. 93–99.
- Bazzano, L.A., Serdula, M.K., Liu, S. (2003). Dietary intake of fruits and vegetables and risk of cardiovascular disease. *Current Atherosclerosis Reports*, vol. 5(6), pp. 492–499.
- Chan, D.S., Lau, R., Aune, D., Vieira, R., Greenwood, D.C., Kampman, E., Norst, T. (2011). Red and processed meat and colorectal cancer incidence: meta-analysis of prospective studies. *PLoS One*, vol. 6(6), p. e20456.
- Craig, W.J. (2009). Health effects of vegan diets. *The American Journal of Clinical Nutrition*, vol. 89(5), pp. 1627S–1633S.
- Davey, G.K., Spencer, E.A., Appleby, P.N., Allen, N.E., Knox, K.H., Key, T.J. (2003). EPIC-Oxford: lifestyle characteristics and nutrient intakes in a cohort of 33883 meat-eaters and 31546 non meat-eaters in the UK. *Public Health Nutrition*, vol. 6(3), pp. 259–269.
- Dinu, M., Abbate, R., Gensini, G.F., Casini, A., Sofi, F. (2016). Vegetarian, vegan diets and multiple health outcomes: A systematic review with meat-analysis of observational studies. *Critical Reviews in Food Science and Nutrition*, vol. 57(17), pp. 3640–3649.
- Etemadi, A., Sinha, R., Ward, M.H., Graubard, B.I., Inoue-Choi, M., Dawsey, S.M., Abnet, C.C. (2017). Mortality from different causes associated with meat, heme iron, nitrates, and nitrates in the NIH-AARP Diet and Health Study: population based cohort study. *BMJ*, vol. 357, p. j1957.
- Katzmarzyk, P.T., Reeder, B.A., Elliot, S. Joffres, M.R., Pahwa, P., Raine, K.D., Kirkland, S.A., Paradis, G. (2012). Body mass index and risk of cardiovascular disease, cancer and all-cause mortality. *Canadian Journal of Public Health*, vol. 103(2), pp. 147–151.
- Lopez, H.W., Leenhardt, F., Coudray, C., Remesy, C. (2002). Minerals and phytic acid interactions: is it a real problem for human nutrition? *International Journal of Food Science + Technology*, vol. 37(7), pp. 727–739.
- Lynch, S.R., Cook, J.D. (1980). Interaction of vitamin C and iron. *Annals of the New York Academy of Sciences*, vol. 355, pp. 32–44.
- Nelson, M., Poulter, J. (2004). Impact of tea drinking on iron status in the UK: a review. *Journal of Human Nutrition and Dietetics*, vol. 17(1), pp. 43–54.
- NHS Choices, (2015). Red meat and the risk of bowel cancer. [Online] Available at: http://www.nhs.uk/Livewell/Goodfood/Pages/red-meat.aspx [Accessed 8 January 2018].
- Weaver, C.M., Proulx, W.R., Heaney, R. (1999). Choices for achieving adequate dietary calcium with a vegetarian diet. *The American Journal of Clinical Nutrition*, vol. 70(3), pp. 543s–548s.
- World Cancer Research Fund International, (2017). Colorectal cancer. [Online] Available at: http://www.wcrf.org/int/research-we-fund/continuous-update-project-findings-reports/colorectal-bowel-cancer [Accessed 8 January 2018].
- World Cancer Research Fund. Red and processed meat and cancer risk. [Online] Available at: https://www.wcrf-uk.org/uk/preventing-cancer/what-can-increase-your-risk-cancer/red-and-processed-meat-and-cancer-risk [Accessed 8 January 2018].

MINDFULNESS

- Hammons, A.J., Fiese, B.H. (2011). Is Frequency of Shared Family Meals Related to the Nutritional Health of Children and Adolescents? *Pediatrics*, vol. 127(6), pp. e1565–e1574.
- Piet, J., Hougaard, E. (2011). The effect of mindfulness-based cognitive therapy for prevention of relapse in recurrent major depressive disorder: A systematic review and meta-analysis. *Science Direct*, vol. 31(6), pp. 1032–1040.

MINDFUL EATING

- Wasink, B. Kim, J. (2005). Bad popcorn in big buckets: portion size can influence intake as much as taste. *Journal of Nutrition Education and Behaviour*, vol. 37(5), pp. 242–245.
- Smith, M.A. (2015). *Calm* (New York: Harper Collins).

SLEEP

- Ayas, N.T., White, D.P., Manson, J.E. Stampfer, M.J. Speizer, F.E., Malhotra, A. Hu, F.B. (2003). A Prospective Study of Sleep Duration and Coronary Heart Disease in Women. *Archives of Internal Medicine*, vol. 163(2), pp. 205–209.
- Chang, A.-M., Aeschbach, D., Duffy, J.F., Czeisler, C.A. (2015). Evening use of light-emitting eReaders negatively affects sleep, circadian timing, and next-morning alertness. *Proceedings of the National Academy of Sciences of the United States of America*, vol. 112(4), pp. 1232–1237.
- Institute of Medicine. (2006). *Sleep Disorders and Sleep Deprivation: An Unmet Public Health Problem*. (Washington: National Academies Press).
- Gallicchio, L., Kalesan, B. (2009). Sleep duration and mortality: a systematic review and meta-analysis. *Journal of Sleep Research*, vol. 18(2), pp. 148–158.
- Hirshkowitz, M., Whiton, K., Albert, S.M., Alessi, C., Bruni, O., DonCarlos, L., Hazen, N., Herman, J., Katz, E.S., Kheirandish-Gozal, L., Neubauer, D.N., O'Donnell, A.E., Ohayon, M., Peever, J., Rawding, R., Sachdeva, R.C., Setters, B., Vitiello, M.V., Catesby Ware, J., Adams Hillard, P.J. (2015). National Sleep Foundation's sleep time duration recommendations: methodology and results summary. *Sleep Health*, vol. 1(1), pp. 40–43.
- National Heart, Lung, and Blood Institute. Sleep Deprivation and Deficiency. [Online] Available at: https://www.nhlbi.nih.gov/health/health-topics/topics/sdd/why [Accessed 8 January 2018].
- The London Sleep Centre. Professor Adrian J Williams FRCP DIPAASM. [Online] Available at: http://londonsleepcentre.com/professor-adrian-j-williams-frcp-dipaasm/ [Accessed 8 January 2018].
- Tosini, G., Ferguson, I., Tsubota, K. (2016). Effects of blue light on the circadian system and eye physiology. *Molecular Vision*, vol. 22, pp. 61–72.
- Williams, A. Why do we sleep? [Online] headspace.com. Available at: https://www.headspace.com/blog/2015/04/24/why-do-we-sleep/ [Accessed 8 January 2018].

INDEX

ACKNOWLEDGEMENTS

This book would not have been possible if I did not have such an incredible team of creative people around me.

First of all, I want to thank my publisher Yellow Kite for believing in the message of The Food Medic from the very start and continuing to help me share my passion with the world. A special thanks to my publisher Liz Gough for saying yes to my very first book proposal, which landed on her desk while I was still at medical school, and now to my second. Also to my editors Tamsin English and Natalie Bradley for helping me to streamline my thoughts and focus my vision while writing this book.

To my dreamy shoot team: Ellis Parrinder, Abi Hartshorne, Jordan Bourke, Fiona Giles and, of course, our resident mascot Frank the bulldog. I have honestly never enjoyed a shoot as much as I have with this book shoot. The process felt so natural, effortless and very creative – not to mention all the laughs we had and the gorgeous lunches we shared. To my glam squad, Roberto Silva and Benjamin Ip, thank you for making me feel so natural and so glamorous all at once.

To my literary agent Carly Cook, and my management team, Jonny McWilliams and Laura Johnson, or, as we have come to call ourselves, #TeamSass. The relentless work you put in behind the scenes does not go unnoticed and I am grateful everyday to have such a team of ambitious people, and wonderful friends, who have my back.

To my mum and my sisters. You have always been my number one supporters and celebrate even the smallest of wins with me. Thank you for being there through the best and worst times. I love you more than I can possibly put into words!

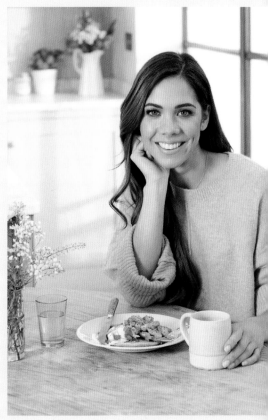

To dietitian Anita Beckwith for working so incredibly hard to complete the nutritional analysis of the recipes and offering her expertise on diabetes and dietetics. You really helped to add something special to the book.

To all the experts who proofread their relevant sections of the book: Dr Megan Rossi, Jennifer Low, Jenny Rosborough and Michael Wong. Your opinions and advice were invaluable in writing this book and I have learnt so much from you.

Finally, to you. My reader. Thank you for investing in this book and investing in The Food Medic. I hope this book helps you to fall back in love with food and feel excited to get back in the kitchen and start cooking. I hope that this book encourages you to ditch the diet philosophy and instead fully embrace food for all the goodness and nourishment it can offer you. After all, food really is thy medicine.